Change Your Mind:
Lose Weight

An Original Holistic Weight Loss Approach for Women

Sandrine Baptiste
Rhonda Tremaine

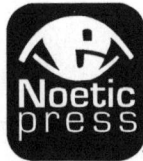

Noetic press TM

Hazlet, New Jersey

Change Your Mind: Lose Weight
© 2011 by Sandrine Baptiste and Rhonda Tremaine.

Cover/Interior Designer: Ian Tremaine

First printing, August 2012.

Library of Congress Control Number: 2012946982

ISBN: 978-0-9858647-0-5

We dedicate this book to our first families, especially our mothers and fathers who raised us and made this physical journey possible.

Mostly, we dedicate this book to our children—Aimee, Ian, Eric, Sydnee and Malcolm—who represent an emerging generation and who we are sure will take the ideas we provide forward.

We thank Ian Tremaine for his exceptional work in designing the ENoetic logo, the interior design of this book, and his patience and perseverance in the creation of a beautiful cover that we all truly love. We thank Eric Tremaine in advance for his forthcoming work on the book trailer. We know it will be brilliant.

We thank Brenda Dunne, not only for reading this book and writing a review, but also for sharing her knowledge about the publishing industry and offering encouragement.

A special thanks goes to Gina Krawczuk and Kat Masterson who volunteered their time and expertise to reading and fact checking portions of this book to ensure its integrity. We thank Debra Clement for editing the legal disclaimer, which enhanced both its accuracy and flow.

We especially thank the significant others in our lives—Dwayne Boatman and Todd Tremaine—who have through the last year and a half understood the enormous time commitment this project required, and supported our efforts in numerous ways.

We thank the random strangers we stopped in bookstores who provided us with the opinions that aided our marketing strategy and fueled our enthusiasm. They all without hesitation unknowingly participated in the creation of this work.

We spoke to many people—too many to name—and we have been supported by our Facebook friends, our physical friends, our relatives, our Twitter followers, and our clients, each of whom has provided invaluable insights and inspiration and for that we are grateful.

But most of all we thank spirit, a force that prompted us to take on this project in the first place, removed obstacles along the way to keep us on a steady course, and infused us with the energy to make the completion of this book a reality.

CONTENTS

PREFACE

Dear Reader,

Gratitude, joy and excitement, coupled with uncertainty and faith, are the feelings that are going through me as I embark on this journey with you. I am a teacher and coach of noetic principles. I am just like you but my perception of the world definitely differs from yours. We are all different. We each experience the world in a unique way. We express ourselves in feelings, and not just thoughts, as we bring our inside world to the forefront to connect with other human beings. Any psychologist will tell you that feelings are at the crux of all authentic experience. So we try to connect, but sometimes there is a disconnect.

Think of emotions as a language. The power of words is different when you speak in your native tongue or in a foreign language. I know. I am French. When I translate my thoughts to English, they are not nearly as engaging or impactful as they would be if I communicated in my first language. Similarly, your inside emotional world does not translate exactly what you feel when you convey your emotions by speaking about them. In fact, this disconnect is so pervasive, and so important, it is in part why I wanted to write this book. Emotions are key, but this book does not represent a weight loss program principled on psychology alone. Instead, it is a holistic response to the issue.

This book has always been inside me. From an early age, I knew I would be a purveyor of knowledge, and I also had an inner knowing that my teachings would materialize in the form of a book. As a child, I would think to myself that one day I would write a book, even though I did not know what it would be about or even if

I was really serious about the prospect. That was before I was fluent in English, prior to my coming to America, and long before I met my co-author.

I was a young psychology student when I first came to America fifteen years ago. I only planned to spend a year abroad, but plans change, and I am still here. Throughout much of those years, I dedicated myself to developing a teaching platform to share what I know. I was excited when I found the coaching model, a strategy that appears much more efficient than any counseling psychology paradigm I knew. Through the coaching model, I am able to help clients to connect the dots between their inner and outer worlds.

When you are doing what you love, you know it. Coaching my clients and seeing them soar has been great, but something was still gnawing at me: I never did write that book. I began to get to work on that missing piece, and then I met Rhonda Tremaine, my co-author, who has been an effective translator and collaborator on this project. We wrote this book because we could not do anything else. We had to do it. Not to take anything away from the effort expended, but this book practically wrote itself. We simply drove the train. The tracks were already in place.

I knew I would write a book, and I did. I achieved that child's dream and it feels wonderful. And that is how life works, and that is how your life will work—just like that—if you change your mind.

Oh, and you *will* lose weight too.

Sandrine

November, 2011

INTRODUCTION

If you are like most dieters, you are probably flipping through the pages of this book and wondering if you will have to count calories or restrict the types of food you eat. You are wondering if there is a gimmick. You have already either read about or attempted most every diet out there, and you think to yourself that calorie counting or food restriction does not work. You are perhaps already enrolled in an exercise program or belong to a fitness center, but you are thinking about quitting because you feel you are just spinning your wheels. You may even feel healthy and eat relatively well, but the weight never comes off. You are tired of the struggle. After all, your efforts have yielded moderate or temporary success at best. What can this book really do for you?

This book will provide you with a better understanding about weight loss that will lead you to naturally embrace a lifestyle consistent with the maintenance of a perfect weight. That is, when you are doing everything right for your body, the pounds will fall off, and your body will in its wisdom, naturally reach a healthy size. Think about it. People do lose weight and keep it off. Everybody knows someone who has accomplished this feat. But when we think about our own inability to lose the pounds, we usually focus on the excuses that have kept us from our goals as opposed to the solution. This is not surprising. People use defense mechanisms like rationalization, to temporarily feel better. Rather than really looking at a situation objectively, they come up with explanations for why they did not achieve their goals.

Ask yourself: Do you *really* want to lose weight? You might say you do, but you also come up with a multitude of reasons that support the idea that you can't. From the notion that your metabolism is too slow to the idea that you don't have the time to change your eating habits, you conclude that your present dilemma is inevitable. The repertoire of excuses is part of your defense, but if you keep reading this book, you will learn how to end these detrimental practices.

You are probably skeptical about this program because nothing has worked for you in the past. But the reality is that if you really change your mind, you will change your weight. How do you change your mind? Reading and understanding how your body works, stepping away from the subjective embrace of your weight loss plight, and engaging in a reasonable amount of exercise, are activities that will each contribute to shifting your thought patterns. This book will also give you the tools to manage your weight, but don't think of *Change Your Mind: Lose Weight* as a diet book. Think of it is a book that will help you to achieve optimum wellness and also help you to maintain that wellness throughout the course of your life.

You will begin by making healthy food choices and engaging in exercise, but implementing changes—tweaking your exercise routines, incorporating new foods into your diet, and adding activities like meditation—is a lifelong process. You will not be doing the same thing year after year, or even month after month. Your body changes as do your needs, and of course, if you did the same thing over and over again, you would be totally bored. In fact, boredom is one reason why many diet and exercise plans fail. The secret to lifelong success is flexibility, not rigidity.

We offer two plans to get you started on the path to wellness. The first is an easy to use portion control strategy that does employ the calorie counting approach. It allows you to make food choices within guidelines that you set. The other plan is less structured and helps inch you toward maintenance. The latter nutrition-based strategy makes use of powerful psychological tools included in this book along with your intuitive insights. Which plan should you choose? You are the navigator of your life so you will decide which plan to try first, but we do help you to come to a conclusion with a short quiz provided in Chapter 8. First, read both plans. Compare and contrast the components to help you decide where to begin, but do realize that you cannot make a mistake. Both plans are rather simple to implement and you can always change your mind later.

Whichever plan you choose, rest assured that starting to eat healthier does not mean your choices will be limited. For example, you can go to a social event and not feel restricted on either plan. Of course, it is obvious that you will not eat whatever you like in vast quantities, but by the time you are well into this program, gorging on fattening foods will be the last thing on your mind. As your stomach shrinks, and you become accustomed to healthy eating, you will naturally choose your foods wisely, so when you go to that party your mind will be more on who is on the guest list than what is on the table. The fact that food obsession will take a back seat to your actual life does not mean you will not enjoy food. In fact, you will probably enjoy food more because you will not be thinking about dietary restrictions. You can go to restaurants and experience the freedom to choose what you like. For example, you may go to a restaurant, enjoy the salad, eat half of your entrée, and then share a chocolate flambé with your partner, and not thwart your goals an iota. How do you manage that?

The ability to make largely healthy choices interspersed with a taste of the more fattening fare comes from knowledge, experience, confidence, and the ability to always make educated decisions. You will be able to reach that point if you read this book and follow the program. You can indulge once in awhile and it need not cause guilt or a desire to diet stringently. You never will think that you ruined your diet, primarily because you are not on one. That point should be emphasized: this is not a diet. It is a plan that culminates in a rewarding and comfortable lifestyle. When you make food choices thoughtfully, you will not feel guilty over a small indulgence, and there is nothing to sort out afterwards. You will always be on track because all that you do within this program is a process, and not an end in itself.

HOW TO USE THIS BOOK

There are two parts to this book. The first part engages you in the philosophy of the program, and the second part provides you with its practical aspects. It is important to read everything in Part I before going on to Part II. This program is not about just putting a diet plan into action. It is about getting mentally ready for a noetic journey. So take your time reading the material. After you absorb the information in the first part, go on to the second. Then do the exercises and take the quiz. The exercises will prepare you for the implementation phase. The results of the quiz will uncover your preferences to help determine which plan best suits you.

As you read through the book, you will have insights that will be important to you as you implement the techniques. A blank page is provided after each chapter for making notes. Alternately, you may want to purchase a notebook to record insights and perform the written exercises. Either way, it is helpful to keep a record of what you learn along the way.

You may find that you want to re-read the first portion of this book after you begin the plan, and this is something we encourage. By reading the first part again, the messages are reinforced and you will probably have new insights as well. Remember, changing your weight is a process and not a diet fix. You can't fail.

Good luck to you as you begin your journey, one that will assuredly be replete with greater awareness, revelations, and increased self-knowledge. When you embark on weight loss in a conscious manner, and understand how your body works, you will become further aligned with your soul's purpose, so while you think you are just losing weight, you are doing a whole lot more.

Part I
Understanding Your Mind, Body and Soul

CHAPTER 1

THE MIND:YOUR
CENTRAL CONTROLLING UNIT

The mind is where it all starts. It is the missing link in the quest to develop a recipe for ultimate wellness. You may think that working out at the gym and making better food choices will help, and while you are correct in that assumption, the problem is that such knowledge does not necessarily lead to motivation. Such knowledge does not provide you with the impetus to get off the couch and exercise and to continue to do so until you are at a healthy weight, nor does the knowledge steer you to the produce aisle in the supermarket. You need something more. Finding out about yourself and getting on the right track will help you to develop the motivation to eat and exercise properly. Willpower alone will not work. Altering your habits without being mentally on board will not work. You need to understand the tools available to you so that you can cognitively overcome obstacles that prevent you from losing weight.

Your mind is a machine, a computer. Like a computer, it has memory, where you can store information and retrieve it at will. However, unlike the information stored in a computer, human memories are often tied to emotion. When you smell a pot roast cooking, your memories may take you back to the kitchen when you helped your mother cook dinner as a young child. When you eat bakery cookies, you may recall a time when you went to a party and saw a cookie that was neither store bought nor handmade. Such recall often occurs at a subconscious level, but the memories tend to push us, at least in these instances, toward certain food choices. You may even realize that you are eating due to an idealized childhood remembrance and refer to the gooey macaroni and cheese, or the meatballs smothered in spaghetti sauce, as comfort food. Eating comfort food seems natural, and a part of the human experience, but its occurrence is more akin to a pre-programmed event than to a conscious choice. Sometimes, this same phenomenon, which is attached to childhood, is associated with more recent memories.

A woman may pick up a chocolate caramel cookie bar, for example, and become immediately enamored of the blend of flavors when she takes the first bite; she enjoys it so much that she buys another bar the next day. She soon purchases a large bag of mini chocolate caramel cookie bars and keeps them in a dish at home, reasoning that she will just eat a small bar, but she ends up eating about six each day, and sometimes she finds that she has eaten the whole bag. She begins to talk about her weakness: the chocolate caramel cookie bar. It becomes a habit, but each time she indulges in the taste of this candy bar, it brings her back to the very first bite when she fell in love with it. This candy tastes so good in part because it helps her to relive the memory of that first bite when she felt good. She thinks she just likes the taste of the candy. However, she is not using her sense of taste as much as she is engaging in the emotional reward of the act. Therefore, while she thinks she is engaging in a human sensory experience, her mind is really acting more like a computer. By eating the candy, she is activating a memory from an earlier moment.

It does make sense to view your mind as a computer because

in part it helps to explain habitual behavior. A computer functions in a certain way—the same way—every time, no exceptions. The human mind also works in a certain way, and it is inextricably linked with the brain. If you've ever witnessed television drama brain surgery, you realize that there are different functions attached to different parts of the brain. With some surgeries, the patient stays awake in order to guide the doctor as he touches different areas of the brain. Each of those areas has a unique function. There are four lobes and each is responsible for different activities such as speaking, moving the body, and solving problems. In fact, your brain has some connection with every part of your body. When someone loses a limb, the brain does not always recognize the loss, and instead perceives the arm or leg as still attached. This example of the phantom limb illuminates the importance of the brain. If we feel as if we have an arm attached when we do not, it is the brain prompting the sensation. The brain is *that* powerful.

The brain has been described as containing a jelly-like material that includes neurons, which communicates through chemical and electrical signals, in order to reach different areas of the body. The brain is an intricate piece of equipment, again, much like a computer. The brain is the center of thoughts and of directives to other parts of the body. Simply, the brain tells the body what to do. It works in such a manner that it affects both emotions and thoughts. Many things can change brain chemistry, including the thoughts that we think, but obviously, other factors enter the picture as well. Because substances can affect our brains, and our thoughts, we also have to look at everything we ingest. Everyone has seen a child who after consuming too much sugar begins to behave badly. The behavior is likely stirred by a chemical process and not related to the environment at all. Similarly, antidepressants work on the brain's neurotransmitters and elevate mood. While we have some control over what we think, we must realize that it is our powerful brain chemistry that is largely responsible for our moods, and the chemicals it contains affect our thoughts. Conversely, what we think affects our brains.

The brain contains billions of nerve cells. In fact, we are born with a certain amount of neurons that will see us through a long life. These nerve cells, or neurons, die throughout our lives. If you think that billions of neurons are not enough, and worry about causing the death of the original cells, new research suggests that we are able to create new connections. The implications of this research are vast and it is reassuring to know that our bodies are always adapting.

The neurons do not actually physically touch one another, as there is a synapse, or gap, between each of them, but in the complexity of nature, the neurons do eventually get their messages across. Neurons contain axons and dendrites. Most neurons have a sole axon that facilitates the transmission of electrochemical material to the next neuron. Dendrites—a more complicated and branched form of material--also allow for the transmission of electrochemical impulses but carries the impulse to the inner core of a single neuron. Thus, the neurons have a method of embracing the substances within their core, as well as the ability to send messages.

The neurotransmitters aid the cause and eventually, the neurons are able to provide the communication necessary for proper functioning. Neurotransmitters do facilitate communication between neurons, but exactly how thoughts affect neurotransmitters is unclear. While there is much discussion amongst scientists on this topic, some theorists maintain that thoughts do have an effect on neurotransmitters. If in fact that is the case, then what you are thinking certainly matters. Your thoughts affect your brain chemistry.

Your Thoughts

Every thought you think, and every food, vitamin or drug you ingest, potentially has an effect on your brain. Your thoughts affect how neurotransmitters react, but it is important for you to understand that it is impossible to trick your brain into behaving a certain way by using affirmations alone or by forcing yourself to think in a particular manner. Your heart must be in it. That said, thoughts do not only affect how the synapses fire, but they affect the choices people make. When people think good thoughts, they tend to make better decisions in respect to what they put into their bodies. This is common sense. When you realize that your body needs good fuel rather than junk food, and you have the chemical balance that helps you to make those choices happily, you will end up at your perfect weight. Simply, it is easier to make better choices when your mind is in a positive place.

Some estimates suggest that we have tens of thousands of thoughts each day. Perhaps you are only conscious of some of them as you ignore most of the things that pop into your head from seemingly nowhere. Some of these thoughts are pleasant, but often your inner critic emerges. You may recognize that some of these thoughts are related to guilt or desire or anger. The thoughts are also seemingly random in nature, something equated with the Buddhist concept of Monkey Mind. This concept holds that you go from one thought to the next, always thinking about the past or the future, and not really focusing on what you are doing right now. You may be working and trying to concentrate on the latest sales figures, but then a thought comes: "I forgot to take my suit to the dry cleaners" or "I hope the bus is not late tonight." Random thoughts—worries, fears, desires—creep into your consciousness and have the tendency to trip you up. In fact, Monkey Mind exacerbates the tendency for human beings to think negatively, to experience random thoughts, and to delve into areas better left untouched. Monkey Mind is the critical mind that chatters incessantly but does not help to improve your life. Also, it is random in nature and does little good. When you allow your thoughts to move about uncontrolled, you will likely end up with thoughts that do not serve the goal of weight loss.

Another point is that most of your thoughts are "re-runs" or a thought that is not new. You may watch a re-run of a television show occasionally, but your thousands of thoughts each day are incessant and those re-runs—unlike what you mindlessly watch on TV-- can thwart your best attempts to manage the way you think. You might obsess about something for days, only to find that another thought comes along to make you think that what you were worried about yesterday is inconsequential, because what is bugging you now is so much more important. For example, you may have a big pimple on your forehead and it really bothers you, but when you receive a phone call from a physician stating that your mother is in the hospital, you suddenly stop thinking about the pimple. Along the same lines, there are thoughts that come into your consciousness once in a while, but they are repetitive. Perhaps every time you put on a pair of jeans, you think the same thought: "These pants are too tight. I have to lose weight." Unconsciously, this translates to feelings of worthlessness. With the same underlying emotion, you might go into the bathroom and think: "I forgot to buy toothpaste. I can't believe I forgot to pick it up at the drugstore!" You are berating yourself for something human. You ate too much. You forgot to purchase a toiletry. So what! You might have these types of conscious thoughts six times or more over the course of three days. When you do finally get the toothpaste, you will not play that thought in your mind again until you run out. Of course, you play similar tracks when you run out of garbage bags, or shampoo, or milk. This is just an example of what you do every day. You have a lot of thoughts in your mind. Most of those thoughts are re-runs. You tend to see these as just thoughts, but you are often not aware of the emotions to which they are attached.

Your Monkey Mind tells you that it will take a long time to lose the weight, that you will never get back into that black cocktail dress, and that you will never attract the partner of your dreams because of your appearance. The list goes on and on. When you last attempted to lose weight, did negative thoughts stop you? If so, it is because the unleashed monkey had done a number on you. The only way to get past this problem is to become familiar with your thoughts and their underlying meanings. Realize that what you think actually affects how you feel, and subsequently how you act. If you are feeling negative emotions because you believe that your diet is doomed, you will go ahead and eat another piece of cake, or you will skip the workout. When you have a negative mindset, nothing seems to matter. You believe that you will fail no matter what you do. The chatter in your head tells you that your actions do not make a difference, but the truth of weight loss is that every bit of activity counts, and that your food choices will ultimately determine whether you are successful in achieving your weight loss goals. After reading these concepts, you can probably now see how changing your mind can help you to change your weight.

It is important to understand how your mind works, and to be able to get a grasp on your thinking, rather than just making a decision to lose weight. When you try to will yourself to do something, you are ironically relinquishing control. Forcing yourself to take action might be fine for a few days, or even for a few weeks, but inevitably, you will succumb to a craving, or you will begin to question your resolve. The loss of the will to continue on the path is inevitable and it is why people say that dieting does not work. While you consciously force yourself to go on a diet, there is an unconscious part of you that questions your actions. Eventually, the monkey you so thought you had under your thumb escapes and the negative thinking returns. How do you get into the mode of losing weight without succumbing to the wrath of the Monkey Mind?

The answer is simple. You have to change your mind. While this is the case, the process of altering your thinking is not so simple. How do you change your mind? First, you have to understand how the entire mind works, and not just how your thoughts emerge. You must take a step back and see your mind objectively. This is not the mind you think you have. It is a mind of great complexity, aligned with myriad beliefs, thoughts, memories, desires and imagination. Yet, everything that enters your mind is sifted through a veil of perception, so what you witness is processed differently than for anyone else having the same experience. That is, there is no objective reality and you perceive things differently from anybody else. In order to get to know your thoughts better, simply question all of your thoughts as they arise. Do this as often as you can, and you will see a difference in your life.

When you examine each thought in such a way, you are the driver, and not the monkey. That is, the thoughts do not control you. A simple example is that you think the following thought: "I have never been successful on a diet in the past." Is the thought true? It just may be, but the truth of the matter is that even if it is—you have not been successful at losing weight in the past—this negative thought has the ability to fester and multiply and continue to creep into your consciousness in other forms. Before you know it, you are also thinking: "I can't lose weight" or "I am worthless." By challenging each thought that enters your consciousness, you are well on your way to reducing the impact of Monkey Mind. This process is very empowering. Simply, you do not take all of your thoughts seriously, but rather, you just notice them, and then transition them into a state where they can actually help you.

To take the example of the negative thought "I have never been successful on a diet in the past," you realize that you have not been able to lose weight, ever. Of course, this is a fact, but it need not lead to a conclusion that you will never lose weight. Most of our thoughts fall into one of two categories, which are thoughts about the past, or thoughts about the future. In this example, you think that you cannot lose weight in the future because you have never lost weight in the past. This is not a fact. It is a belief. A negative belief will stop you every time. To change your mind, you have to challenge your beliefs.

Beliefs: The Ties That Bind Us

Beliefs are the foundation of the thought process. After all, everything you have taken into your consciousness in the past has been evaluated and either integrated or rejected. People collect beliefs throughout their entire lives. We can all relate to the notion that people in a family do things a certain way, or believe in some of the same things. This is because we live with the people in our first families, at least most of the time, and we often share DNA. There is much about our lives that intertwine with family members including religion, culture, an aptitude for certain hobbies or careers, and even superstitions. The idea that you will have bad luck if you break a mirror, or that you are doomed if you inadvertently step under a ladder, are beliefs that are based on stories that have been handed down, but they have no merit. Other beliefs come from a mere chance occurrence. You develop a belief not based on something from your family or culture, but from a random event. An example is that one day, your morning begins badly—you spill orange juice all over the table, you have a screaming match with your kids, you misplace your keys—and your thought is that this is going to be a bad day. And guess what? You're right. You believe it is going to be a bad day, and this gets into your consciousness and the bad day manifests. This is what is referred to as a self-fulfilling prophecy. Yet, the bad day starts with a simple belief. Where did the belief originate?

A belief can come from anywhere. Again, it can come from family, but it can also come from a mere statement that someone says in passing. You may have seen someone become very angry when he spilled coffee all over his white shirt. You witnessed the event and empathically keyed into his emotions. The look on his face is cemented in your mind. He muttered something under his breath that suggested because of the event, it is going to be a bad day. You hear it, hardly give it a thought, but when things start going wrong for you after you spill a drink, you ponder the original comment, at least unconsciously. Thus, once a man spilled coffee on himself and he concluded that it will be a bad day, so every time you spill something, you believe it is going to be a bad day. These types of ideas and opinions have been accumulating throughout your life from different places. When you begin to believe some of the things you think, then you begin to live by these thoughts and integrate them as rules.

Challenging beliefs can mean the difference between

failure and success. Yet, it is important to remember that not all beliefs are erroneous. Many beliefs have validity. There are things that are true and healthy and good for you. If you believe that you can succeed, that is a good thing because it is true. The trick is to eradicate the negative beliefs that are holding you back, which is why it is important to examine them first. What do you believe? What is truth and what is a falsehood? How do you know what is true? Ask yourself a question and then listen for a response. The response may not necessarily come in the form of words. It might be a feeling that yes, what you are thinking is true. The truth will feel good. It will feel as if it is right. Sometimes, you are unsure, but more often than not, the indecision will not be based on a gut feeling, but rather on your intellect. Your intuition comes through your veil of perception but you can trust its message. It is coming from a pure source as opposed to your ever-present, always thinking mind. It might take some time to fine tune your inner knowing, but it will come if you keep practicing.

It is important to connect with your inner self because faulty beliefs can thwart the weight loss effort. If you believe that you can't lose weight, you won't. Why attempt something that is impossible? If you knew that no matter what you did, you would never lose weight, you would never try. Of course, while that point is obvious, what is not so obvious is that you have placed limits on yourself by believing something that simply is not true. You believed that you cannot lose weight, but the truth is that you can. Catching thoughts and challenging them before they become beliefs is integral to controlling Monkey Mind. When you no longer believe something, thoughts related to the belief will fade. Getting rid of faulty beliefs is just the beginning. Implementing new programming is also necessary to change your mind.

How To Change Your Mind

Remember the idea that human beings are capable of introducing new connections to the brain, something that was thought impossible years ago? Neuroplasticity is associated with the notion that brain pathways can change in reaction to stimuli. We think positively and see positive results. We eat healthier, and then we begin to crave foods that are good for us. Neuroplasticity is a concept that supports the notion that our thoughts, our environment, and our actions can change our brains. And because the brain controls every inch of our bodies, this is wonderful news. You may be able to change your brain function by acting and thinking differently, as well as by making healthier food choices. And while this is certainly applicable to creating wellness, it is also applicable to a number of things. When you talk about doing something new, implementing new habits, and thinking new thoughts, you are creating new connections in your brain, and this is happening beneath the surface.

Changing your mind is an inside job. It means that you have to be proactive in working on yourself with the recognition that you can change your brain communication system, and this in turn changes how your entire body functions. When you change your lifestyle for the better, you will be changing your emotions, and it will be that much easier to eat well and exercise. If the scientific theories are correct, you may be able to alter the way that your neurotransmitters react by thinking different thoughts. In fact, antidepressants create a better feeling state in the same way. Food can also act to alter the chemistry in your brain.

Think of your mind as an electronic device that contains numerous apps or applications. We are essentially programmed to do certain things. You might be programmed to wake up and make eggs and bacon, and then at three o'clock eat an ice-cream cone, and you think that it would be difficult to alter these habits. After all, your afternoon snack is non-negotiable and you are just not the fruit and cereal type. You research various diets and conclude that the meal plans will not work for you because they exclude the foods you love, and you cannot fathom having to live without them. Of course, you own the apps that are set to a certain way of eating. You are the one who programmed them, and so you are in control. You can change the apps.

Obviously, if you can change the apps, you don't have to keep living the same way. You simply have to delete the bacon and ice cream apps and download the cereal and fruit apps. You can change your habits in this way. Further, you need not—nor should you—change your apps all at once. In fact, altering your lifestyle too drastically will likely lead to a meltdown. The phenomenon where your dietary habits change for the worse after you ditch the plan is often referred to as diet backlash. The idea of diet backlash is that you make changes too drastically so you never integrate the good messages, and you eventually give up. Rather, you plunge ahead, having been caught up in the excitement of visualizing yourself several sizes smaller, but you have not really thought things through. Crash dieting, or making any sort of drastic change, will not serve your brain chemistry well. It is important that you not make radical shifts.

When you change your apps, think small. With only slight variances, you will lose weight healthfully without suffering, and you will see results every month. How do you make small changes? If you are waking up and eating a big breakfast of eggs, bacon, orange juice, toast and butter, and you are resistant to changing this pattern, you need not discard the habit completely. You want to eat healthier, and you also want to shed pounds. If weight loss is your desire, you must either eat fewer calories or exert more energy, whether you are doing so purposefully or not. Simply substitute some of your typical selections with a healthier choice. A fix for the breakfast just noted might be to have one egg with turkey bacon and whole-wheat toast with a cholesterol lowering spread. Keep the orange juice because it's healthy, but if you water it down, you will reduce your calorie intake even further. This same principle may be applied to a number of situations. Do you usually order a soda and a large buttered popcorn at the movie theater? Instead, choose a diet drink and a small popcorn without the butter. This small change could save you hundreds of calories.

Changing your apps is not difficult. It is a process that is associated with making small changes. You are reprogramming your computer. You are rewiring your brain. When you make a decision to eat cashew nuts and an apple as a snack, instead of potato chips and dip, you are utilizing a new app. When you do this consistently, you are in the process of changing the app for the long haul. This change may not be permanent. Just like you buy software for a trial run that stops working in 30 days, you can try the change for a short time. You eat a healthy snack and realize that it tastes good, so you stop buying potato chips altogether. You do this voluntarily because you have found a delicious treat that makes you feel better, but when you make this a conscious choice, you are changing the app, at least for a while. Again, like a computer application, things change. Apps become obsolete. After a month, you may not want to see another cashew nut. No one likes to do the same thing over and over again. So you change the app again. Next, you might want to try apricots or yogurt or cheese. Change is good, and changing your apps will help you to thrive mentally and emotionally as you lose weight.

Recent authors have recommended that habits, or eating some of the same meals over and over again, can help to cement a healthy lifestyle, but such tactics can actually lead to failure. Eating the same things over and over again, or living with the diet mentality, is boring. Further, deprivation can shake loose even the most dedicated dieter. When you are eating what you like, but not varying your repertoire, you will grow tired of the same old things, and this can lead to an abandon of your plan. You may suddenly decide to get rid of all your new apps, and download the old ones again just because you crave change, but that would be detrimental.

Thinking of your brain as a computer containing apps helps you to understand how your mind works and how you can change it. You learned that changing your mind is really not that difficult. At this point, you may be wondering how the apps you programmed can be so easily altered when your brain is like a computer. In other words, if your brain is programmed a certain way, it seems that it should just continue on that path forever, barring some significant intervention. The ability to change apps just seems too easy. But the human mind is probably more flexible than you realize. This is because while the analogy of the brain to the computer works, it only goes so far. You are more than a machine, so altering your apps is possible, but there is something larger than your brain and your mind that enters the picture. The inexplicable thing that works behind the scenes is your inner self.

The Inner You: Your Foundation

You are a multi-dimensional being. You are human, of course, and you know that you have a fully functioning body and mind. You can feel things, sense temperature and taste food. You can grasp onto a tangible item and use it. You can run, you can paint a portrait, and you can sing. You can do a number of physical things, but what is inside you is what holds you together. Your foundation—what makes you "you"—is your spirit. You as a human being, and you as a spiritual being, live in a world where you have a multitude of responsibilities. You work and take care of your home. You worry where the rent money will come from, or whether you will have to endure another root canal. You worry about the safety of your children. When you think about it, the stress is unnecessary because what you are worrying about is temporary. You know this intellectually, but it is hard for us to really integrate this concept. It is difficult for us to see these important elements of life as unimportant. On some level, we know that we are spiritual entities first --an entity that knows no physical death and goes on forever— but our problems seem very real. The understanding of who we are does not change us automatically. Still, we change a little bit at a time. Soul relationships become more important than the electric bill we can't pay because the former is something that lasts for eternity, while the other represents a temporary difficulty that is part of the challenges of living life on Planet Earth. Once this knowledge is fully integrated, we are changed forever. While this is by no means an instantaneous change, it is true that understanding your spirituality is the foundation that helps you to change your perspective.

As you go through life, you gain both book and experiential knowledge, and while one can say that the latter is purer, both converge to provide you with the opportunity to change. You may ask a question and then find the answer in a book, or you may have an experience and talk to someone else to validate it. As you embark on your spiritual journey, you are changing, and that changes your perception. Your perception is the lens with which you view life. It is your perspective, your point of view, but while that is the case, your perception changes over time. When you get in touch with your inner self, your perception will change immeasurably.

Your soul or higher self is an intangible but important part of yourself that actually plays a role in your success. Although your "inner you" plays a critical role related to behavior, you are still a physical being that relies on the body to function according to the laws of science. Again, your brain contains neurons that communicate with the rest of your body, and you can program your mind. By changing your apps, you will make better food choices. Of course, when your soul is in congruence with those changes, the results are extremely powerful. At that point, you will lose weight with great ease.

If you cut calories and exercise more, you will lose weight. However, if you are not fully on board, the changes you make will likely not last. You may go through the motions—counting calories and hitting the treadmill—but at some point, your enthusiasm will fade. That is why it is so important to align your mind with your spirit. This will help you to become fully engaged in the process. The change is something that happens over the course of months so it makes sense to change your habits gradually. Move towards a healthy lifestyle and you will see results every day in terms of vitality, satiety, and of course, weight loss. One of the most important things to remember is that this is a process. You probably gained weight over a long stretch of time, and it will take time to lose it, but if you follow this program you will never suffer nor feel deprived. And once you are at your perfect weight, you will probably agree that the process has been worthwhile. Not only will you be thinner, but you also will experience radical growth in respect to your soul's journey.

Understanding your soul is different from understanding the

physical functioning of the brain. We know the mind is attached to the brain and a bit about how it works, but the soul is more illusive. Perhaps the only scientific research on the soul was conducted early in the twentieth century by Dr. Duncan MacDougall where he concluded that the soul weighs 21 grams. That the soul can be thought of as tangible or quantifiable is interesting, but Dr. MacDougall's body weighing activity is not considered scientifically valid. Also, even if the soul has actual weight, its essence and experience differs for everyone. More recent research shows greater promise. Dr. Sam Parnia has been engaged in a project that attempts to determine whether near death experiences are fictions of the brain, or true spiritual events. If he is successful in this quest, there could be scientific evidence of the soul's existence in the future.

Understanding our soul's mission and connecting to it can help us to lose weight. You do have a soul, and it plays a role in weight loss, but how it is integrated really depends on how much you want to explore it. This is not something that can be rushed, so this understanding and connection will come over a period of time. In the mean time, understanding how your body and mind works and how to make changes is key. However, your imagination will accelerate your progress as you make these gradual changes.

Imagination: The Product of the Soul

Changing the apps sounds like something you do on a computer, and while you can systematically alter the apps that exist in your mind, it really is not done the same way as it is done on a computer. After all, you are a human being. The computer is just a metaphor. Your mind is still a mystery even though you know how your brain (the hardware) and your mind (the software) work together. You know what imagination is, but have you used it lately? When you were in kindergarten, your teachers probably prompted you to use your imagination to draw pictures or create models out of clay. You were likely encouraged throughout elementary school to create things from your imagination. But as you grew older, you were less encouraged to use your imagination and were instead guided toward more practical endeavors. Of course, while this would not yield a room full of robots, it does make Jack a very dull boy.

Your imagination can help you to change your mind because it allows you to visualize, think about things in a different way, and to create a future that you want to move towards. Your imagination takes you beyond your senses and into a world that you make. You decide what will happen to you, and when you realize that you are able to use your creativity to change your life, you will begin to see what is possible. Have you ever pasted a picture of your head on the body of a model you cut out of a magazine? It seems a silly thing to do, but it actually helps you to see yourself differently. You don't need to make a collage to see yourself in a new light. Visualize how you will look when you are thinner. You may not be able to do this immediately but your new self will emerge in your mind's eye over time. This is one benefit of having a human mind. You can create your world, and that includes a world with a slimmer, happier, more vital you.

The use of pictures, vision boards, mind movies, and guided meditation helps people to clearly decide on a goal. For weight loss, you might want to create a movie in your mind where you think about how you will look after you achieve your weight loss goal. If you have already been at this desirable weight, you might want to find a picture of yourself and post it on the refrigerator or keep it by your desk. The more you see yourself the way you will be, the more you will believe that it is possible. And as you know, believing something is an important component for eventually making your desires materialize.

Spend a few minutes each morning, just after you wake up, thinking of your new body and how you will be feeling and what you will be doing. You might want to picture yourself in a bathing suit taking a morning swim in the ocean, then warming your feet in the sand before finally rinsing off. While you visualize yourself in this manner—experiencing an active, healthy life where you look and feel great-- also experience the feeling of pride and happiness as you no longer struggle, but are able to live the life you always desired.

Perception: What Makes You Unique

You learned about the intrusion of unwanted thoughts or your Monkey Mind, but everything that comes into your consciousness through your senses comes through a veil of perception. The exciting part of this is that everybody's perception is different. Your perception is in part attached to your DNA, your personality, your inner knowing, and how your senses work. If you are blind or deaf for example, your sense of touch, taste and smell will be heightened, but if you are a visual artist, you may perceive the world aesthetically through your eyes where other senses become secondary. Your perception enters the picture because it plays a role in how the information from the outside world, and from your inner core, converge to form thoughts, and again, the thoughts you think have a dramatic impact on how you feel and ultimately what you do. When you use your imagination, you do so through your own unique perspective.

Some words of advice are to question your negative thoughts, eradicate them, and use your imagination to replace them with new ideas. Once you are able to do this, you will alter the way you perceive the world. The question is not whether perception affects your thinking or whether your thinking affects your perception because both are true, but rather, what will you do to change your mind? The ideas to come from this chapter—questioning every thought, eradicating faulty beliefs, changing your apps, getting in touch with your inner self, and using your imagination to create your future— will help you achieve weight loss success. And all of these things are attached to your mind and how you think.

Thinking is More Than You Thought

When you started this chapter, you may not have anticipated reading about your spirituality or your perception of the world. While this first chapter does address the mind, and compares it to a computer, you have also been exposed to the notion that the mind and spirit are connected, and that your perception makes you uniquely you. As you read through this book, you will be introduced to the science of emotions and you will learn more about spirituality and how your perception makes all the difference.

But first, in the following chapter, you will be introduced to your physical body, which is not detached from your mind and spirit, but is also—like having a mind—a uniquely human experience. That is, as we walk around, we do so in physical armor and it is that armor that protects us from the environment, but what is important to acknowledge is that the physical armor is what we are trying to change here. So understanding exactly how your body works is vital.

Notes

CHAPTER 2

THE PHYSICAL YOU: YOUR EQUIPMENT

This chapter is dedicated to the physical you, the part of yourself that is skin and bones, and vital organs and veins. The physical you refers to everything about your body that you can touch as well as parts that are seemingly out of reach. While we are all spiritual beings having a human experience, it is the physical body that encapsulates the spirit and is so important to maintain. Your body is the vehicle in which you are taking your life's journey. Without proper maintenance, and occasional repair, your journey may be marred by unexpected incidents that hinder your career, your relationships, and your daily routine. We strive so hard to get everything done, and in the process, we put our bodies last. We may reach for a corn dog and a soda and vow to eat better tomorrow, but not putting ourselves first results in neglect over time. The incidents of putting off doing what we know is right in order to take care of immediate concerns add up. Soon we are engaged in bad habits that seem hard to break.

The purpose of this chapter is to show you how your body functions, how complex and interconnected your operating systems are, and how easy it is to really understand what is going on beneath the surface. By exploring the systems, you will obtain the information necessary to view yourself in a different light. As you may have already concluded, changing your mind really matters.

It is what this book is about. When you see what you are made of, you will see yourself differently and that transition is integral to changing your mind. When you change your mind, you will begin to put yourself first and that will make all the difference.

In order to understand how your physiology affects your life, a tour of the human body is in order. You may know some of the information already, but you may not have integrated it as part of yourself. You likely do not see your body as a piece of equipment. Rather, you conduct your life by using the body, making the parts move as the environment demands, and just going through the motions to get from place to place. By engaging in mindless behavior, you have not accepted the reality of the situation. That is, your body—like your car or your washing machine—is a machine in and of itself.

While you may understand the information intellectually— you know your teeth chew your food, you know that your stomach processes the food after it makes its way through the esophagus -- you have not altered your mind in such a way as to make the information an unconscious part of how you live. Once you can take a step back from your body, and see it more objectively, you will also begin to view eating and exercising in a different way. Food will become the fuel for your machine and exercise will become the way you maintain your machine. When you change your thinking, such a paradigm shift will take you away from the emotion that is likely tied up in some of your negative daily food choices as well as your excuses to forgo exercise.

Other information will be brand new and will help shed light on the machine you so very much want to take care of. From a spiritual perspective, your body is the machine that allows you to go through this particular corporeal existence. Without it, you might end up in a blissful afterlife or in another incarnation, but the truth is that you will not be able to experience all that life has to offer right now. You might think you are a cerebral or spiritual person who is not in need of help from the physical world, but the truth is that it is only through taking care of your body that you will be able to thrive in the present life experience. It is an integrated approach—melding mind, body and spirit—that really works.

What you will learn by the time you are finished reading this chapter is that there is a new way to look at your body. You will see your body in terms of functionality, but you will also have an appreciation for the marvelous apparatus that it is, how complex it is, and how all of its systems are interconnected. To really understand the concept, think of your body as a perfectly functioning machine. From the top of your head that houses your brain to your ears to your arms and legs, each part of your body has a different job. Think about what each part of your body does. For example, you might first think about the fact that you can read this book so your gift of sight is functioning, and then you may realize that you are able to smell flowers with your nose, and you are able to taste food with your mouth, and so on. As you think about everything your body can do, it becomes apparent that the body is a marvelous, living thing that when functional, operates in a perfect manner.

Your body in fact is just a machine with a number of systems that make it run, much like an automobile. Now, detach from your emotions. Stop thinking about your body for one moment, and think about your car. Imagine that your automobile needs repair. Would you avoid the mechanic? Of course not. You would welcome his advice, even though you might not want to pay the bill. Would you blame yourself for not taking the car in sooner, or believe that if only you had gotten an oil change one month earlier you would not be in this situation? No, you do not fret because you simply take the car in and forget about it. You will either pay the bill or get another vehicle. Of course, the analogy does not work so well when talking about the human body because unlike a vehicle, we only get one body, and you cannot take your body to the shop and leave it there while you go do something else, at least not in this human experience. Why are we using the automobile as a comparison?

It is true that your body is much more important than any vehicle, but you have experienced emotions related to your car. Yet, the emotions you experienced in respect to your vehicle is certainly not as intense as worrying about having a heart attack or fearing cancer, and that is exactly why you need to look at your body objectively. If you get away from it, you will be able to understand it better. Ironically, this experience will also make it more personal, and it will make taking care of your body more rewarding. Maintaining objectivity is difficult to accomplish, but by detaching from thoughts about things that could go wrong with your physical body, you will actually be helping to maintain it.

While you may be aware of your entire body that is composed of myriad organs and numerous systems, many of you still haven't a clue as to how everything comes together. This is why it is important for you to understand the systems that make up the physical body. Some people know everything about how their cars run so when they go to the mechanic they know whether the mechanic is skilled or trying to rip them off. People who do not know what goes on under the hood are at a disadvantage and are more likely to be emotional when the car breaks down. Have you ever heard of someone talking to their automobiles, saying things like "please start", when the starter is completely gone? Someone who is mechanically inclined will be inquisitive, and will realize that only a small repair is necessary and either change the starter, or take it to a trusted mechanic to do the work. When you know about cars, you are more likely to make better maintenance and repair decisions. The same is true for your body. When you understand how it functions properly, you can take a step back and see what is going on when it begins to malfunction. A "car guy" knows which fuel to use, and how to perform the oil change, as well as how to drive it for greatest efficiency. Similarly, when you know how your bodily systems work, you will be able to exert energy in an efficient manner, and take in nutrition to best serve its function.

A Tour Through Your Body

While systems are important, it pays to start the tour of the human body with an examination of the single, solitary cell. The cell is a tiny particle. You have many cells within your body. In fact, your entire body is composed of tiny microscopic cells that divide and attach themselves to one another in certain ways. They migrate. They multiply. They are each attached to various areas of expertise as they transform into nerve cells, blood cells, bone cells or become one of a number of other specialty cell types. But the cells are not running around rampant. They are not thrown around in a chaotic mess. Rather, the body in its systemic wisdom creates an orderly situation that sees the cells behave. The cells converge to create the marvelous figure that we have come to know as the human body.

In all, your body is comprised of eleven distinct systems but they are interrelated. The integumentary system is a good place to start. It represents your skin, which is comprised of several layers, and serves to protect the body from the outside world. You could not survive without your skin. People who have experienced fires and who have suffered from burned skin throughout most of their bodies rarely survive. And while you know about your skin largely because you take care of it with sun tanning products, moisturizing creams, and repair injuries with ointments, you may not know that your body also has something all around it—much like a thin stocking—and it is called fascia. Fascia is technically connective tissue and it exists around the perimeter of your body just below the surface of your skin, and it also goes through it to connect every part of you. It surrounds your internal organs and all of your muscles. It is something that is physical but barely visible. The fascia, and the whole of your skin is important, but what you are perhaps used to thinking about in terms of your physical body is your skeleton. The skeletal system in fact does provide the underlying structure for your physical shape.

The skeleton starts with your skull and includes your teeth, and it makes its way down through your throat, chest, hips and legs. Of course, you are familiar with skeletons, a favorite decoration at Halloween, but it is the structure of our bodies that is most solid. Its purpose is multitude. It enables us to walk, to raise a glass with our hands, to bend and turn around, and it also serves as protection for our vital organs. The skeletal system makes up an important part of our bodies. It gives the body shape and form on some level. It dictates height. It provides the body with structure, and of course, the skeletal system runs through the entire length of the body.

The muscular system, similar to the integumentary and skeletal systems, comprises the entire length and width of the body. You may be familiar with this system if only because many personal trainers reference the specific muscle groups when they provide instruction. While we think about our arms and legs as having numerous muscles—and they do—we often forget that our facial muscles are important, as they allow us to convey emotion. Without these, such as the orbicularis oris muscle, nonverbal communication would take a completely different turn and we would also have a hard time consuming food. And of course, we cannot forget our abs. There are a multitude of books and exercise programs that solely target the abdominal muscles. The muscle groups described provide just an inkling of the relevance of this system. The muscles all over our bodies are important.

We are aware of our skeletal muscles, but we also have smooth muscles that operate beneath the surface, and further, it is important not to forget about the all important heart muscle. You may be thinking, isn't the heart part of the circulatory system? Clearly, it is, but systems overlap. There are smooth muscles found in numerous systems, and of course, the heart is associated with the circulatory system as well as the muscular system. The lungs also play a role in terms of cardiovascular health, but they too are integral to the proper functioning of the respiratory system. Each system is vital, but they are inextricable with the other systems of the body.

The circulatory/cardiovascular system includes veins, arteries and the blood that runs through it, from your head to your feet. It is literally the lifeblood of your body. The respiratory system takes in oxygen, and it gets rid of carbon dioxide. Think of your respiratory system as an air converter. It uses the air that you breathe, and then it expels what is not needed. The digestive system begins with your mouth. When you eat, you chew food by using your teeth and your facial muscles, and then you swallow. You may not think about where the food goes, but it takes a rather interesting trip down a long tube called the esophagus. When food is digested, it churns through the stomach, but over the course of time, the food is transformed and ends up in the small intestine, and then the large intestine, and finally eliminated. However, the nutrients from the food do enter the bloodstream. Knowing how food travels through the digestive system, and how important it is to nourish your body, does provide you with a sense that what you eat is important. Similarly, what you drink matters, and this brings us to the urinary system.

The urinary system that consists of the kidneys, the bladder and the urethra, eliminates urine, which contains waste materials. The system also helps to regulate fluid. Your circulatory system is related to blood pressure, but the urinary system regulates the amount of water contained in the blood, and this is associated with blood pressure too. That the urinary system only eliminates fluid and does little else is a misnomer. All the systems work together. Another example is the nervous system. Similar to the circulatory system that allows blood to flow through your veins, the nervous system links everything with nerve fibers. Nerves are found everywhere, even in your brain, and it facilitates communication throughout the entire body.

The endocrine system regulates your body in a number of ways through the production and release of hormones. Hormones are important to the proper functioning of everything from metabolism to sexual activity, and it has an effect on mood. Throughout their lives, women rely on certain hormones. These hormones are implicated in the reproductive system as well, which again signifies an overlap. Finally, the immune system helps our bodies to avoid a variety of illnesses. The eleven systems are always working, and when even one of them malfunctions, an illness may result. That our bodies work in this intricate fashion gives rise to a sense of awe. It is rather amazing not only how the body functions, but that it often functions well, particularly when we take care of it.

Integrating the Information

The body is seemingly mysterious, but scientists have been studying it for quite some time, and while mysteries remain, physicians have a good grasp on how to take care of it. Yet, it is not enough to visit a physician and follow her advice. We must know our bodies to make the best choices. Rather than do that, we all too often ignore it. In fact, we often act as if our heads are separate from our bodies. We are so in our minds most of the time that we forget we even have bodies, but we do have bodies and they are in need of care. The importance of the physical body should be emphasized. You intrinsically know this, which is probably why you long for a good-looking encasement for your functional systems. But even if you are not craving a beautiful form, recognize this: we need the body to take us to the places where we use our brains, so understanding how they function is key to feeling in control. In fact, you *are* in control. Although the human body may be illusive to those of you who have not taken Anatomy and Physiology in college, the cursory tour of the human body you have just taken is sufficient for this understanding.

Now that you have read about each of the systems, you probably feel more connected to your body already. However, you might want to delve deeper into some of the systems. Reading and understanding how your body functions objectively can help you to see yourself in your fully human experience. You may decide that you want to gear your diet to address a certain medical condition, or you may want to tweak your diet to gain more energy. With the advice of your physician, and a clear understanding of your body's functioning, you can alter your diet to improve your health. Similarly, knowing how your body works is key to understanding weight loss.

It is your body from which the weight is vanishing, so knowing how it operates makes the experience more personal. Understanding the body objectively is key to developing the motivation to give it proper care, and part of the necessary attention relates to eating and digestion.

When you eat, it is not a situation of garbage in/garbage out, where someone eats junk food, and it goes through the body and is expelled. Rather, whatever nutrition can be extracted from the food is utilized by the body, and when you think about that, you will begin to realize that whatever you put into your mouth counts. You may be familiar with the expression "a minute on the lips, a lifetime on the hips," but that is an expression tied to the diet mentality. It is made to prompt you to think that if you eat something it will end up as fat on your body. While it may be true that eating a treat that contains upwards of 400 calories could conceivably be consumed in sixty seconds, and it will cause you to gain weight, that sort of thinking drives you to the refrigerator. It prompts feelings of guilt, and causes you to question your choices. So when we are examining the functions of the body, the revelation that prompts you to eat healthier generally takes time. Such information is not meant to cause tension. Rather, you might grab an apple and realize that it has a lot of fiber and that is good for your digestive system. You compare it with a candy bar that has perhaps four times as many calories and a lot less fiber. The candy bar may contain high fructose corn syrup and a number of ingredients you hardly recognize. You know the apple is natural. It comes from a tree. The candy bar, on the other hand, is made in a factory and wrapped in paper. Which is better for your body?

You knew that the apple was better before you read about the workings of the body, but now that you are beginning to integrate an objective view of your body as a marvelous machine, you may gravitate more towards foods that are closer to nature. Now, if you still prefer the candy to the apple, don't think that anything is wrong with you. The process is gradual. Learning about your body brings you to a place where you can objectively make decisions about your fuel, but even after you have integrated the material, you may sometimes choose the candy. And there is nothing wrong with an occasional candy bar, but there may be an explanation for what drives your poor choices. Part of your system includes emotions, and the emotions are often responsible for a continual focus on unhealthy food. When you gravitate towards this type of eating often, something else is going on. The next chapter provides you with a unique way of understanding your emotions so that they don't control you.

Notes

CHAPTER 3

THE EMOTIONAL YOU: BETTER DECISION-MAKING THROUGH EMOTIONAL INTELLIGENCE

By now, you have a better idea about how your body works. You know that it contains intricate systems. You are also probably beginning to realize that if you take care of your body—the marvelous machine that allows you to run, jump, think, and breathe—you will be healthy and the excess weight will vanish. While caring for your body often results in weight loss, the result is contingent on your completion of the steps required to achieve the goal. That is, thoughts do not translate to action automatically because emotion gets into the picture. You may think you want to try losing weight, but then emotions come flooding to the surface and stop you in your tracks. Your emotions may bring up fears and thoughts of past binges, or they may create a movie where you try on clothes that do not fit, or they may prompt a myriad of other insights that really do not serve you well. These examples are aligned with thoughts, but they are filled with, and fueled by, emotion. In order to go from thinking about weight loss to doing something about it, you have to apply this program to your life, a program that will supply you with the motivation and tools you need to succeed. Additionally, you must be willing to tackle those emotional blocks that have stopped you from becoming your best self. Understand that the emotional attachments you are carrying are stopping you from losing weight. It is only through dealing with these heavy emotions that progress on this program is possible.

Before delving further into the concept of emotions, how they are holding you back, and what you can do about them, it is important to look at the subject. What are emotions exactly? How do they work? Why do we have them? Emotions are equated with our feelings that are associated with a state of body and mind. Emotions are often triggered by thoughts, but they are attached to physical and physiological processes. The butterflies you feel in your stomach when you are near a new love interest, or when you are about to take an important test, is part of the physical aspect of emotion. You know it is physical too because sometimes it is not your thoughts that provoke emotion. For example, if you are in the premenstrual phase of your cycle, or you have suffered a broken arm or leg, emotions flood forth. Hormones affect your emotions as does a physical injury. When it comes to emotion, there are two kinds of triggers: internal and external. Internal cues have to do with your thoughts and your physical experience. External triggers are events in which you find yourself. You may be driving behind someone who is going slowly or you feel the ground shake and realize that an earthquake is about to occur. In such instances, you will feel negative emotions such as anger or fear. Although emotion is attached to internal and external cues, there is another dimension, and that is the spiritual aspect of emotion.

In the bestselling book *Molecules of Emotion*, the well-known pharmacologist Candace Pert suggests that while western society does not often acknowledge the connection between energy and emotions, many ancient and alternative healers think otherwise and refer to this energy as chi or prana. Our connection with source does open a gateway for emotion to be triggered. When you have a feeling about something, that feeling may come from something beyond this physical reality. Seeing a future husband or wife across the room and knowing that this will be a perfect match is inexplicable. You see a complete stranger but have a feeling that something will come of the relationship. It is an emotion that might be explained through psychology, but another explanation does lie in the realm of the unknown.

Emotions serve a number of purposes. While they may help us select our life mates, they also help us to avoid pain. In *The Gift of Fear*, Gavin de Becker suggests that we have an inner knowing that can help us to not only predict whether a violent attack is imminent, but also to help us in our response to it. Our inner knowing in part is attached to our emotions. Emotions act as an alarm. You wake up during the night and feel something is not right. Then you hear someone banging around the house, so you immediately sit up and dial 9-1-1. Your emotions by that time have gotten the better of you. Your heart is pounding, your mind is racing, and your hands are shaking, but you are relying on your emotion to lead you to the right action, and your emotions triggered by that inner knowing will give you the right advice every time. Clearly, emotions are more than chemicals that create chaos in our lives. Yes, emotions are sometimes negative, but they often serve a positive purpose even if it is to get us to sit up and take notice of a situation. The situation could be that you are being burglarized, but it could be about the fight you had with your mother in law, or the worries you have about the longevity of your job. When it comes to emotions, many different events can act as a trigger.

Emotions and Overeating

You probably notice that people who go on crash diets, or even people who diligently follow healthy eating regimens, often regain the weight they initially lost. Likely, you have heard of this happening time and time again. There have in fact been scientific studies that link attempted weight loss with ultimate weight gain. The phenomenon is well known, and has often been referred to as yo-yo dieting. What happens is that unwanted pounds return when you do not do the necessary work to hone your coping skills. When you lose weight without engaging in the preparation required by the process, you are not likely to have long-term success. In other words, if you merely lose pounds through diet and exercise, but do not do the inner work or deal with your emotional eating triggers, you could resume your negative eating habits. Why does this occur?

Some overeaters indulge in food because it distracts them from their daily lives. They eat a lot, think about food, obsess about restaurants or cooking, and build a life where eating takes center stage. They think about other things of course, but food is very important in their lives. One might think of it as a form of entertainment because it is a distraction that does take up a lot of time and is sanctioned by society. When people socialize, they usually do it over food, whether it is at a house party or a restaurant. Being a "foodie" is actually trendy, and cooking has become a form of entertainment as evidenced by the growth of The Food Network. There is nothing wrong with this if overeating is not part of the scenario and in fact, there are many thin people who like gourmet fare. Yet, this focus on eating suggests that food indulgence is an important part of life. The problem with elevating food to a significant level of relevance comes when people have health or weight issues, and consume more calories than their bodies require.

If a woman does focus much of her attention on food, and is eating more than she should, this is most likely because she developed eating strategies that helped her to cope with uncomfortable emotions. Unfortunately, while this allows her to cope with difficult emotions in the short term, it does not serve her well over time. Not only will she have gained weight as a result of this way of living, but she also will have missed out on the personal growth that is possible when real emotions are experienced. That is, if she learned to cope with difficult emotions while they were emerging as opposed to using food as a distraction, she would have experienced life at its best. It is hard to believe, but personal growth can be both difficult and marvelous at the same time. If only she knew this, she would have been able to overcome her negative coping strategy and taken life head on.

What Happens When You Ignore Your Feelings

Emotional eating may be viewed similar to a state of denial. When you eat, you are holding your life together. You work, you clean your home, you take care of your children, you go out to dinner with friends, and you think you are building the good life. Everything is shiny and clean on the surface, but if you dig deep, you might find that your emotional state does not match what you show the world. It is more likely than not that you are burying some of your feelings by engaging in emotional eating. When you do this, you hide what is really troubling you. For example, you may be experiencing guilt or shame or anger. You do not tackle the issues that have triggered those feelings so they go unexplored. Perhaps a talk with a counselor or even a discussion with the person who prompted those emotions would clear the air. When you ignore interpersonal relationships or fears or worries, they get buried. Even if emotions are recognized, they are not dealt with, so the result is anxiety that is quelled through overeating.

Emotional eating is a reason why many people are overweight. However, that is only one reason. While many use food as a drug, others simply never learned how to eat properly. If you are in the latter camp, where perhaps obesity is a family problem, you may not think this chapter is as relevant for you as for someone struggling with her feelings, but it is still important for you to understand your emotions. When you lose weight, you will likely experience emotions you did not know you had simply because the experience of losing weight is an emotional one, but also because you will be feeling the emotions you thought you buried a long time ago.

As you lose weight, and tone your body, your shape will change. You may need to buy new clothing. People will treat you differently. If you prefer to remain on the sidelines, you will be disappointed. There is probably no better way to garner the attention of others than to sport a slender physique. Many of you have purposely been hiding from the world, but losing weight will force you to participate in places you once feared and with that, there is personal growth.

In 1943, the psychologist Abraham Maslow presented a typology suggesting that if a human being has not met her basic needs, she would not care about meeting higher level needs, such as safety, love, esteem, and actualization. When using Maslow's hierarchy of needs, it is quite obvious that food is at the base of the pyramid, because it is only when you have satisfied your basic needs for food, water, and so forth, that higher level needs may be met. If you cannot breathe and you are experiencing gnawing hunger, you will not care about your relationships. You will only care about keeping yourself alive. However, when your primary functions are restored, you will begin to think about safety. You may feel good, but you also begin to consider the future. Alternately, when you are overeating and focusing on unhealthy fare, you distract yourself from your real life. You likely make more compromises than you should. You settle for what life throws at you rather than making your own choices. Instead of indulging in life's pleasures, eating becomes your most significant pursuit. While eating is something to be enjoyed, the overemphasis is misplaced. When you eat too much, how can you know if you are meeting your basic need for food? You are not paying attention to nutrition. You are eating to cope, and in the process, you ignore sound nutrition, you don't sleep enough, you may not drink enough water, and you are probably are not taking care of yourself in other ways. By thinking about food differently, you will be able to enjoy delicious meals and actually lose weight in the process.

You may think that talk of food obsession is an exaggeration. After all, you may be already eating in a fairly healthy way and your life seems to be working. However, once you start losing weight, you will begin to re-examine your life. When you feel balanced in terms of meeting your basic needs, you may go out and look for a better job, or you may look to improve your relationships. Now, an overeater may have plenty of food in her stomach, but she is not doing everything she can to fulfill her needs for safety, or for intimacy, or for esteem. The problem is that when you overeat, you are out of balance. You need to balance this first needs level, and as anecdotal evidence suggests, once you eat the right amount of food, and really take care of your body, you will feel better about pursuing your dreams. Your self-esteem will naturally rise. You will begin to explore self-actualization as your physical condition improves and you will move up the needs hierarchy. In effect, your journey to lose weight not only helps you to fulfill your basic needs, it helps you to climb out of the rut you were in when you were just getting by.

Your New Journey of Feeling

On a practical level, the weight loss process comes with temporary ups and downs, but it is one that will lead to a better life. However, it is good to know what you will be going through as you head towards your goals. Again, the idea that you might have been hiding not only suggests that you will need to climb out of your comfort zone, you will no longer be invisible. When you walk to the grocery store, or pick your children up from school, you may be noticed. When you lose weight, you might do better at work or muster the courage to get a new job. You might receive attention from potential suitors. While such outcomes are often desirable, it is still a change, and most changes come with stress and apprehension. Before you lose weight, you might think you would not mind the attention, but feelings of vulnerability or indignation may rise to the surface. When you are smaller in size, you might feel more amenable to whatever is being foisted upon you. Also, when you receive attention simply because you lost weight, you may feel that people like you for superficial reasons. Many emotions are stirred as the weight falls off. Of course, negative emotions—much like all emotions—are temporary. As you lose weight, you will not only experience uncomfortable emotions, but you also will experience positive ones as well, and so while the ride might be bumpy, it will not necessarily be difficult.

Using Your Body as a Shield

On some level, layers of fat offer a feeling of protection, but the truth is that this is just an illusion. That illusion keeps you from dealing with your strengths, your vulnerabilities, and your real feelings. If you feel that you are using your body as a way to separate yourself from people, you may think that this is impossible after the weight is gone. That is, you will not have your size keeping you from meeting other people. When you are heavy, you are more likely to keep to yourself, and are less likely to make new friends or interview for new jobs. You may argue that you have nothing to wear or that you will do something about your loneliness when you finally lose the weight, but when you are at your desirable weight and are in excellent health, you have no excuses to stay home. If you are shy, this could create a situation that takes you beyond your comfort zone.

Another uncomfortable situation is when weight loss prompts significant changes such as the ending of a relationship or a job. When you lose weight, your confidence soars. Self-esteem rises. You feel so good about yourself that you are more likely to examine your present situations and while the result might be divorce or unemployment, the truth is that you were perhaps not as happy as you believed. In other words, when people lose weight, they feel powerful because they are in control of their bodies. They are then ready to tackle other issues in their lives, whether it is an abusive relationship or a dead end job.

On a superficial level, it appears that you are making changes to stroke your ego. Who has not made negative comments about the stereotypical middle aged man who loses weight, and the next thing you know he has a wife half his age? But on a deeper level, the weight loss inspires soul-searching that leads to positive, lasting changes. Further, as you stop emotional eating, you will be feeling your emotions more frequently and on a deeper level. This is good, even though it may be uncomfortable at first. By experiencing your feelings, you will be able to discover who you are and what you really want. You will be moving towards self-actualization, which means that you will begin to fulfill your potential.

People who are obese often eat their emotions and distance themselves from other people. When the weight falls off, they not only have to deal with the emotions they experience during the process—the easy part—but they also have to deal with their relationships, which will inevitably change. They also have to acknowledge the goals that they put on hold. You know the ones: these are the things you tell yourself you are going to achieve once you lose the weight like planning a trip to Hawaii, going back to school, or writing a book. While losing weight and becoming fit might allow you to do the things you always wanted to do, your vision may not come about. For example, if you wanted to travel the world, you simply may not have the funds to do so. Circumstances may not allow you to go back to school. You might fantasize about meeting the partner of your dreams, but that partner has not yet materialized. That weight loss is not a panacea is an idea that may creep into your conscious thoughts, causing you to really consider the possibility that the fat was not the only thing making you unhappy. In fact, it was not necessarily the fat preventing you from enjoying your life. Rather, it was a symptom of a life that was not completely satisfying.

As thoughts come into your head about what you might have not known on the surface, you may feel frustrated or sad, but this is part of the process of change. Your weight was your excuse to feed the status quo, but now that you know your weight is not responsible for putting your life on hold, you have the opportunity to change. Part of the process of weight loss is not just losing pounds, but recognizing what you were not doing with your life, and making changes just a little bit at a time. Of course, emotion—both positive and negative—is something you will have to manage throughout the process of losing weight. It is not something that will be easy, but it is the work that you should have been doing instead of overeating, and while it may sound like a daunting task, the truth is that it is probably the most rewarding part of the whole endeavor. However, because some emotions feel bad, it can be a bumpy ride. Understanding how your emotions work will help you to navigate the unfamiliar waters.

The Science Behind Your Emotions

Your emotions are hashed out in the brain. Yet, it is the sensory information that you take in from your ears, your mouth, your nose, your fingertips, and your eyes that enter the fray, providing information for the brain to process. Sensory neurons send their messages, sometimes connecting with interneurons. The brain participates and determines whether or not a response is required. And while it seems so simple—that the sensory information enters the brain and comes out as emotion—it is really not that simple. It is not a matter of something coming into the brain, being spun around as if in an ultracentrifuge, and being spit out again. Rather, before sensory information enters the brain, you screen it in your own way because your perception differs from anyone else's.

Your perception—which is the programming that is in place—along with your extrasensory perception, instantly weeds through the information derived from your senses. When that data enters the brain, it merges with your thoughts, and emotion is created. Your thoughts are energy, and as you know from reading about the mind, the brain works through the use of chemicals and electricity, so when it takes in this sensory information, it processes it in such a way that the energy culminates in feelings. The emotion that is created in your brain, resulting from what you take in and perceive, is rehashed and released as the feelings you experience.

Pert writes in *Molecules of Emotion* that because there is no objective reality, human beings need emotions to filter the sensory information they receive. We need to make sense of the information in some manner. So, we go into Macys and there is a deluge of merchandise, but we gravitate toward the shoe department, filtering out the men's tie area and the women happily spraying perfume at passers-by. When we get there, we further use our emotions to select the perfect black pump to go with that little black dress. Throughout the journey, our emotions are always on and always working. Yet, the shift in focus is conducted on an unconscious level. Because this is brain chemistry, and the brain is inextricably linked with the body, Pert looks at the physical human being as a mind-body. Indeed, the body is flush with chemical receptors. Our bodies are chemistry sets that are charged by electricity. You already know that this goes on in our brains, but it also goes on in our bodies. We feel the emotions in the stomach or solar plexus. The emotions we perceive from sensory information after it is churned through the brain reaches different parts of the body, and the result is often a mixture of physical feelings and thoughts.

As you can see, your thoughts affect how neurotransmitters behave, and that in turn affects how you feel. An example is the euphoric feeling that emerges after running for a long time. You may not be familiar with this sensation, but it is often referred to as a runner's "high." This happens because the brain manufactures endorphins—a type of neurotransmitter—after your body is under stress for a period of time. While you are running, or doing any extraordinary exercise that places the body under duress, the brain manufactures chemicals to take the edge off. The endorphins help to make the body feel comfortable, but the result is that you feel like you are able to tolerate the discomfort of the continual exercise. In the end, you feel good, and so exercise comes with this extraordinary perk. The body, on some level, is exercising its own wisdom by prompting you to feel good so that you will continue to engage in an activity that is good for you. Another example of brain chemistry changes is aligned with the manufacturing of chemicals during meditation. In such an instance, there is an increase in neurotransmitter activity. By examining the examples of running and meditating—two things that help you achieve your health goals--you can easily see how the brain, the mind-body, or whatever you want to call the headquarters of your physical self, runs.

Your brain is an energy mix of sensations and thoughts that churns out chemicals and these in turn end up as the feelings you experience. Although the process may appear rather cold and objective, the truth is that your perception—a topic for which this book devotes an entire chapter—is what makes your feelings personal. You are more than your emotions, your brain chemistry, or even your feelings. You can control the ruminating thoughts, which in turn controls your feelings, but what is perhaps the most extraordinary observation is that you are not who you thought you were. In other words, now that you know how your body works, and how your emotions work, you probably realize that you are a spiritual human being, who with different thoughts and a different way of perceiving the world, will end up with different feelings. You can change your thoughts, and by doing so, you can change your weight. This knowledge—when applied properly—will result in an improved state of mind, something that will help you to lose weight.

Notes

CHAPTER 4

THE SPIRITUAL YOU: THE POWER IS ON ALL THE TIME

We are all on a spiritual journey. We come into this incarnation not only with different missions to fulfill, but also in different states of readiness. Some of us are on an accelerated path, having recognized the spiritual aspects of ourselves long before we integrated the proper terminology. We may have happened upon spirit through playing with Tarot cards or an Ouija board when we were young, or through continually asking philosophical questions. Brief exposures to spiritual elements throughout life are not accidents. We are all on the path of growth and what we find along the way helps us to cement a spiritual direction. Wherever you are in life, and wherever you are in your spiritual journey, just start the process from there. Start this program from wherever you are. Wherever you are now is all right. It is where you are supposed to be, and it is from that vantage point that you should embark on your weight loss quest.

One of the first signs that you are on the path is that you begin to ask questions about the universe and where you fit in. Your vocabulary now includes terms like "life purpose" and "the meaning of life." Anyone who is searching for something more, and connects with these types of concepts, is beginning to recognize life for what it is, an existence that is just a piece of a large continuum. We are living an Earthly existence, but we are more than what we know on a practical level.

The Energy That Fills You

You are an energetic being. In fact, there is always a current of energy running through you similar to how electricity runs through a television set or a dishwasher. But unlike a household appliance, this type of electrical current is not visible or measurable. You don't go to the doctor and find out how much energy you used, because this type of current is not quantifiable. And, of course, you are a physical being. You are made of skin and bones and blood that exist in a large intricate semblance of systems. When you go to the doctor, he takes blood samples with the use of a needle, and glass collection tubes. He does not use an energy meter like your electric company representative because while there are actually electrical impulses in the body, the energy that is closely equated with your soul is the power that is part of something more that connects all human beings. It is spirit energy that flows through us, and that flows around us, and that serves to connect us. This type of energy differs from the electrical circuits that exist in our bodies and differs from the electricity that generates power to our homes and businesses.

Unseen and nonphysical, this energy is something with which we are all familiar. If you have ever had a creative urge, or a moment of clarity, or have used your intuition, then you know what the energy is like. When you are experiencing it, you are inspired, you feel authentic, and you are excited about the future. And while you can sometimes decipher where the inspiration or the good feelings came from, a specific point of origin is not always obvious. When you are connected to source energy, you feel good. Rather than going through life and being subject to emotional reactions to external events, you can draw on your inner power supply and be able to manage your life with fewer difficulties. Situations and the chaos that is often equated with daily existence will no longer rattle you if you are connected to your inner power reserves. If you are hooked up to source energy, you are less likely to be influenced by life's seemingly random fluctuations. Know that when you are connected to source, you are infused with the same energy that creates worlds. Whatever you do, you can't fail. You are *that* powerful.

By now, it is obvious that your inspiration and creativity are elements that are more than firing synapses and hormonal shifts. While we are thinking and breathing beings, we are more than the compilation of the different systems that make our bodies work. We are more than the electricity and chemicals that travel through our bodies. We are more than the sum of our body parts. We are intelligent beings, and while that is the case, artificial intelligence can never mimic the depth of the human spirit. It is impossible for man to create a human being without the vital extraordinary cells that includes worlds of their own and while scientists can produce clones, they are just assisting a process that already exists. They are using the marvelous cells that are infused with spirit energy.

Connecting to Source Energy

So where is this energy that exists in your body? Why haven't you recognized this current yet? You may have ignored the current because you are busy going to work, going to school, taking care of your children, or just attending to daily tasks like cleaning the house or paying the bills. You probably do get a taste of it occasionally when you go to yoga class or immerse yourself in a hot bath, or perhaps before sleep when you turn off the television and revel in those first few moments of silence before you drift off. To get in touch with your higher self, you have to get quiet.

On some level, you already know how to connect with these deep energy reserves. It is inside of you already, and you connect to it through recognition and stillness. Recognition is important. You have to know that it is in there. Again, you may have stumbled on it by going through the motions. You may have attempted meditation, or you may have experienced a sense of connection without consciously understanding exactly what is occurring. But to consciously explore your inner world takes you to the next level. You have begun to ask questions, but when you ask questions consciously, and with conviction, you are fervently exploring the universe. When you specifically try to connect to your inner world, you are running—not walking—on the path, and that is okay. You are driven by a desire to find answers. You are asking questions now, and while the answers do not come with the same lightening speed as they are sent out, they will come eventually. When you meditate, you are clearing space in your mind for the truth to enter, a process similar to how your hard drive is defragmented. Again, your mind on some level functions like a computer and even though you are a spiritual being, you have to understand how to use your physical equipment.

Your mind enters the equation, but it is the act of dancing with the energy—accepting it and allowing it — that results in connection. To get the sense of this, imagine that you have a small box inside your solar plexus. It is filled with energy. For those who have never tapped this resource before, the energy is dormant—at least most of it—and it sits inside that box. The small box deep inside you corrals and protects the energy until you are ready to utilize it. At that point, when you go within and explore the inner self, you will begin to shatter the borders of the container in which the energy resides. This is usually a gradual process. As you find this spiritual energy and begin to utilize it, the box will begin to deteriorate, and as the box weakens over time, more of the energy will escape and fill your body. Of course, your spirit is not literally in a box, but the illustration does convey a sense that the source energy deep inside of us is always there, and it is always accessible. You just have to allow for it. The energy will seep through the box if you let it, but it is your call. The power source for the box is always on. It is on all the time. You may not recognize it yet, but rest assured that you have this energy waiting to be accessed. The box inside you is full of energy, but much of it is contained until you are ready to use it.

Many of you are in touch with your spiritual side already. You engage in meditation or you have had spiritual experiences that are real and life changing. Others have had some experiences that created leakage. That is, your experiences have whittled holes in your energy box, something that allows your spirit to emerge. Simply, some of the spiritual energy contained in the small box ekes out. You may have been singing in a house of worship when you felt that peace that you have been told transcends human understanding, or you just ended a phone call that seems to have put you in a deep state of relaxation. In the latter example, you wonder if the stranger at the other end of the telephone line was an angel because you feel you have made a spiritual connection. Ordinary experiences can be spiritual because there are holes in the box. For example, an incident occurs and you recognize the incident as being otherworldly. You notice synchronicities and begin to feel differently about the world in general. As you begin to connect with the energy that comes through the box, you ask more questions, questions that lead you to information that helps you to understand what is going on. How much of the leakage is experienced is an indication of how much energy actually fills the cavity of your physical body and is dependent on your current stage of spiritual growth.

Recognizing who you are can be life changing, but it is also important to note that you live on Planet Earth for the moment, and you also are in a physical human body. You experience a range of emotions in your present existence from elation to despair. A spiritual understanding of the universe makes it easier to cope with the difficulties of Earthly existence, but your spirituality is not something that exists just to make your human life easier. It is simply who you are. When you gain a better understanding of the reality of this, you will not only experience joy much more frequently, but you will also find meaning and purpose in your life. You will find that some of the answers to the questions you have asked begin to emerge.

The spiritual journey is after all one that is human too. Sometimes, you will forget who you are and allow yourself to experience states of negative human emotion. Some of these emotions are necessary and desirable because we are human beings and are fully living this existence. An example is that when someone dies, grief helps with the desirable emotional release, something that is part of the healing process, and helps you to cope with the shock of separation. An evolved being knows that death is simply a transformation, but losing a person we have come to know on the Earth plane is an inevitable human experience. The tears of grief translate to how much we have loved. As we go through life, we will experience some perceived negative events, but they are ultimately for spiritual growth.

The spiritual journey is rewarding, but it is a process. Like anything else, change does not happen overnight. Yet, it is worth the trouble because embracing your spirituality and taking it to the next level results in both internal and external rewards. The journey is in itself rewarding but ultimately, the person who you become is equated with confidence, satisfaction, excitement, and abundance.

Spirit: Finding the Real You

The spiritual journey is on some level taking a leap of faith, going on paths you never would have dared, and believing in things you never thought possible. The element of the unknown and speculation about what might occur sometimes stops people from embarking on the path. They keep their boxes closed and when there is a little leakage prompted by synchronous experiences, or insights that come out of nowhere, they fearfully plug up the holes. Then, they just go about their business. They pay their bills, they watch television to fill the time between social and business activities, and they think they are living a happy life. They may even explore their spirituality pragmatically but without actually progressing in their spiritual understanding of themselves. When they do think about the deep questions such as why they are here, or what their purpose is, they are often distracted by their commitments. Keeping busy is one way of never finding out who you are.

Do you want to know who you are? The quickest and easiest way to align yourself with this energy is through meditation. The electricity, or the spirit, is the glue that holds everything together. When you meditate, you get in touch with what is inside and you are able to access your inner world, which is all that is real anyway. Think about it. Do you rush through life going from one thing to another, gobbling fast food that passes for lunch and rushing back to the office, and never really stopping to be still? Do you read books with a running commentary—the chatter in your head—so that you do not fully absorb the material? Are you doing this now?

All that is real is inside of you. You really do not need anything else. Your inner voice will guide you on your path toward personal fulfillment, and meditation is the best way to accomplish this alignment with source energy. Meditation will be explored in the second part of this book where you will be provided with instruction on how to implement a daily practice.

What Does Spirituality Really Have to Do With Weight Loss?

Thus far in this book, information has been relayed about how the body functions. There has been an emphasis on the idea that your body, your mind, and your emotions can work for you, but also how they can work against you. That you understand your systems and how everything is put together is important for successful weight loss. It can help in the development of self-efficacy, something that is important to the weight loss process. Self-efficacy is equated with a belief in yourself. When you are confident about your abilities and the program with which you are working, you will feel more positive, and that leads to motivation. Viewing your body as a machine that needs attention will help you to understand why the food you put into it is so important to its proper functioning.

That better nutrition can improve the way you feel, and enhance your overall health, is old news. Everyone knows that. If it were easy to change from junk food to healthy eating, everyone would just do it. The missing ingredient is of course a belief in yourself, something that leads to proper motivation. If you are more motivated to sit in front of your television and eat brownies than you are to go roller skating or bicycling, you will likely take in more calories than you need. However, if you are motivated to change your weight, and you understand how your body works, you will be more inclined to make better choices. That said, the understanding of the workings of the body is just the beginning. Comprehending the science of the human body helps you to understand what it needs, and it will indeed spark some motivation, but it is the missing ingredient—spirit—that will help you to get to a place where you really care about change. When you are connected to source, you are connected to truth, and then you will feel as if you can do anything. There is nothing more powerful than the truth. When you understand this, nothing else can bring you down.

Start From Where You Are

You are an energetic being, but the degree of your connection is largely determined by how far along you are on the path. What you may not realize is that while we all have different life paths, the speed at which we progress is inextricably linked with our motivation to succeed. It is the part of us connected to source that grounds us, and it is important to remember that the power is on all the time. The electricity that is contained in the little box is always there for the taking. It can be set free. Poking holes in the box over time provides you with a sense of it, but if you are at a stage of your spiritual evolution where you are ready to soar, you will be pleasantly surprised at how quickly you will be able to lose weight.

How can you tell if you are at a stage of development where you can open the box and let your spirit loose? One way is to look inside. Do you feel ready at a gut level? If so, then you are. Otherwise, you would be reading this portion of the book with a lot of skepticism and little enthusiasm. At the same time, if you are not fully on board, it does not mean that this program will not work for you. Any move towards spirituality will help you to change your inside so that your outside will change too. Further, everyone is born to be on a different spiritual path and is ready to make a breakthrough at different chronological ages. Generally, we come into the world as infants, and then grow to be spiritually open children, but our enthusiasm and creativity is largely stifled by the world's respected institutions. We go to school and religious houses of worship. We are taught to believe in certain things. And after we are given the wondrous memories of Santa Clauses and Easter Bunnies, we are told even before adolescence that everything we knew is a lie.

Of course, we are on the Earth plane to do physical things. We are spiritual beings first, but we are living a human experience. Yes, we are spiritual beings, but we are frankly here to get our hands dirty, fall in love, learn reading and writing and arithmetic, and have babies. We are here for many things and we do forget who we are often after the end of childhood. As we age, and particularly as we near toward the end of our human journey—at least in this lifetime—we begin to ask the big questions. We do this earlier perhaps, but with answers ambiguous or unresolved, we get busy and forget to ask again. At some point, many of us recognize that we are no longer able to bury our questions and keep that box closed. The energy oozes out. We begin to gain both book knowledge and experiential knowledge as we read and meditate. We grow spiritually and emotionally, and while we do that, we are getting into a state of readiness to change our outside world.

It is important to embark on your weight loss journey with a spiritual foundation or weight loss will be just another preoccupation. People go through their lives doing things. They have goals to purchase homes, to drive new automobiles, and they save for retirement and college educations for their children. They also want to look good. They go to the salon, have plastic surgery, wear contact lenses, whiten their teeth, and receive Botox injections, but perhaps the most serious flaws they want to correct is attached to their bodies. Everyone wants a perfect body, and part of the equation is to be at a perfect weight. And while being in a suitable weight range is certainly desirable, the truth is that dieting can be a distraction. This is why you need a real transformation, and not a diet. Lasting weight loss comes after you make spiritual progress. Although anyone can lose pounds by eating less and exercising more, it seems that for weight loss success, you need a spiritual solution.

As Your Spirit Soars, Your Body Gets Lighter

You have just learned how important spirituality is for your personal growth. Weight loss on some level changes your perception of who you are. When implemented properly, weight loss is the end result of inner growth. As the spirit fills your body cavity, you become lighter figuratively, emotionally, and physically. The lightness of being is attached to the choices you make, the foods you eat, the thoughts you think and the practices in which you engage. When you make meditation a part of your daily routine, you are putting yourself first. As you look within, you are going down the rabbit hole, but you are doing so with the knowledge that taking these first steps is the best way to not only lose weight, but to live your life to the fullest.

Notes

CHAPTER 5

PERCEPTION: HOW THE MIND, BODY
AND SPIRIT COME TOGETHER

Every person's perception is different. Everyone has his or her own way of experiencing life, but that is good. It is what makes people unique. Like the blanket analogy in the 2004 film *I Heart Huckabees*, we are all connected, but the concept might sound scary because the ego is lost when we think this way. The ego, as used here, is a term that refers to the conscious, rational part of your mind that you see as yourself. It includes your intellect, your personality, and the things you perceive as being aligned with who you are, but it excludes the spirit or who you really are, because it does not go there. The ego lives in the physical world and protects your physical body. It does not concern itself with the soul because the ego divides people, rather than unite them. This is not a bad thing. The ego simply distinguishes you from your brother or your neighbor or your best friend. Your ego defines who you are as an individual human being.

The term ego has a bad connotation, but the ego is connected with your personal identity, and your ego quite frankly wants you to think that you are all there is. This does not mean your ego wants you to think you are alone, but rather, it wants you to think that you are separate from everybody else. Everyone has an ego. People go through life with desires, goals, and a certain capacity to perform.

They have different opinions, different talents, and different backgrounds. The ego distinguishes people from one another. Of course, the ego is not all there is, and you know that. Still, the loss of identity or personhood or ego or whatever you want to call it is a bit frightening. Sure, it is nice on one hand to think that when we die we emerge into a nonphysical existence and become a part of a blissful body of energy, but on the other is the reality of the situation, which is that we want to be individuals. We want to stand out. We do have egos. So on some level, we fight with our desire to belong to this larger energy we know is out there, and revel in our connection to source and the signs we see along the way, but we still want romantic entanglements, we still desire fat bank accounts, and we still long for a sense of physical security. Most of all, we cling to personal identity as if it is the most important thing in the world, but by now you know it isn't.

The knowledge of something more on some level is not always enough to convince us that we can trust what we know, because again, we are physical beings with a psychological makeup that comes with a personality tuned to this particular Earthly channel. We will not easily give up our attachment to our material goals, our relationships, our opinions, or anything that is uniquely ours. When you think that you are just a part of the greater landscape, and you lose your personhood, you worry that you might lose yourself. It is a valid concern, but it is impossible to separate from who you are. Your inner self is perhaps linked with other people, and with the world, and what we like to think of as source energy, but while the spirit is connected to everyone else, parts of your personality are attached to your soul. On some level, your personality is fused with your ego, but it is a part of the inner you too. So you will never disintegrate, you will never deteriorate into nothingness, and you will never cease to be you. Your uniqueness is retained at a soul level, but again, you are still on a physical journey. Right now, you live on Planet Earth. It is advantageous to live a life with all the worldly physical possessions and relationships you desire. As you journey through life and attempt to manifest a satisfying existence, it is your perception that makes a difference.

What is perception exactly? Perception is the filter with which you view the world. Your perception is not your ego. It is not your spirit. However, it is the tool you need to bring everything together. Perception serves a purpose. It is the translator that helps you navigate the world. It is your point of view, or your position in this lifetime. It is the crafted sieve created by you based on your experiences, but it is inextricable with who you are as a physical human being. Your DNA plays a role too. Long before you were born, you were comprised of cells that are attached to strands of DNA that programs who you are. The DNA is associated with a long lineage of ancestors. Your relatives may be a lot like you. You may resemble your parents physically as well as emotionally and mentally. Richard Dawkins coined the term meme to denote the transmission of culture that is handed down from generation to generation. Of course, you identify with your relatives, and with your culture, to an extent, but there is more than this identification. Again, you are not a robot, so your preprogramming, and even the programming you receive as part of your culture or first family, only provides a semblance of a controlling force. The rest of you is that unseen, inexplicable, spirit energy that brings your personality through and also incorporates everything around you. So your perception is attached not only to you as a physical egoic human being, but also to your inner core. Everything converges and through your perception, you get answers, and these answers—as you live your life—become the wisdom that you use to make all of your decisions.

Perception may seem to be an intangible thing that is difficult to fathom, but knowing you have it will make a difference because it explains why you do what you do. People go through life, again, with beliefs and with ideas that are faulty and negative. They may start a diet and then quit while they are actually doing well because they feel as if they are not progressing fast enough. Their innate belief that they have no power, and that they might as well quit now rather than be defeated, gets the better of them. So when a woman thinks that she might as well not go forward with something because of low self-esteem and a lack of a positive belief, understanding that it is her perception that is holding her back can make the difference between success and failure. An example is that Suzie decides to go on a diet, and as soon as she makes this decision, there are many thoughts that come flooding forth: "How will I stay on my diet when I have a wedding in a few weeks? I don't know if I can give up eating ice-cream in the summer. If I go on a diet, everyone will be watching to see how well I do." The thoughts are simply a part of how Suzie perceives the world. They are certainly not facts. Let's question these, one thought at a time.

First, Suzie worries that she has a wedding to attend. Although she wants to look good for the wedding, she fights the idea of starting a diet immediately because she knows she will be faced with temptation down the road. She imagines herself at the wedding. She even has a large dress that is flattering to her figure and she can wear it and look good. She would like to have a piece of wedding cake, and she will not know what else is being served, so it will be hard for her to follow a diet plan. Simply, she feels that she cannot plan in advance, so what is the point of trying to diet? Is this belief reasonable? The idea that she cannot possibly stay on her diet while attending a wedding is not a fact, and it is not even rational. Many people lose weight and attend events. Why might Suzie perceive this situation with stress and angst rather than matter of factly considering the reality of the predicament? There are many reasons why Suzie is upset about future events. It is possible that Suzie had only been on inflexible and stringent diets. It is true that if, for example, Suzie went on a diet where she would not be allowed any carbs, she would have to forgo the cake. Suzie might have also been in the situation before. Perhaps she did not eat the wedding cake, and she regretted the decision. You may be thinking, it is just a piece of cake, but to Suzie it is a relinquishing of her personal power. That is, she sees giving up the freedom to eat cake as a symbol of a lack of freedom in general. If she realizes that her feelings are attached to her perception, she can make a good decision.

An example of a solution to the problem is that Suzie can count calories, and eat whatever she likes by choosing wisely. She can have a piece of the cake, which might be equivalent to approximately 400 calories, and while this might put a dent into her calories for the day, it is doable. She has the freedom to eat the cake if she really wants it. Another possibility is that she need not count calories on the day of the event. She could still start calorie counting immediately, lose weight over the course of a few weeks, and merely not count calories on the day of the wedding. She fears feeling deprived because she already gave up the cake in the past, and does not want to live like that. Of course, she does not have to. And while perhaps that is a simple look at the situation, there is more if she wants to dig deeper. Most likely, what Suzie is really afraid of is that the wedding will cause her to abandon her effort completely. She is afraid that if she eats the wedding cake, she will go out and buy cake the next day, or she may be afraid that she will feel deprived when she returns to her diet. There are all sorts of fears that emerge, but she is letting Monkey Mind get the better of her. This all happens largely due to the way she perceives the world. Otherwise, she would just go to the wedding, maybe eat a few things that are not on her usual plan, and then return to better food choices the next day without a worry. At least, that is one way of perceiving the situation in a more positive light.

Suzie believes that dieting is something to be done where there are hard and fast rules that cannot be broken. Her background is that she comes from a family of heavy people and her mother, Janet, had always been on and off diets. When Janet was on a diet, everyone would grow tired of hearing her talk about how many calories are in each piece of food she ate. Janet would go on extreme diets where she would eat only salads, cottage cheese and diet shakes for months, while the rest of the family would eat balanced meals. Suzie felt that not only were her mother's choices unhealthy, but that they were difficult to follow.

Suzie's background on some level plays a role in how she perceives things. The filter through which she sees the world has a hand in formulating her false beliefs. Her personal experiences also play a role. When Suzie went to band camp, another child called her names because of her size. As a result, Suzie would be very cautious about choosing clothing. Everything she wore was oversize. Although Suzie did not look attractive in dark, baggy clothing, she thought she did, so when she wore something she believed was attractive, she did not worry so much about her weight. Her perception was that everyone believed that she looked attractive, and that she did not look fat. Thus, when the wedding invitation came, Suzie immediately thought about the black dress with turquoise trim she wore to another wedding. It is very roomy, and she even got a compliment on it. She would do her hair in a certain way, and it would give her a sense of elegance. Suzie perceives that she will look good at the wedding. Her beliefs about dieting are further supported by the perception about her appearance. It gives her more ammunition to argue for delaying the weight loss attempt.

Another fear of Suzie's is that she loves ice-cream and does not want to give it up during the summer. She perceives the summer as a fun time. She likes to go to the beach, and her favorite part of the day is buying ice-cream. Again, the idea that she will not be able to eat ice-cream is faulty. It is quite reasonable to eat ice-cream while counting calories. She simply has to make the ice-cream a part of the plan. Today, with a large number of choices—no sugar and nonfat varieties of favorite flavors—and with a typical ice-cream bar being only about 150 calories, there is no reason that Suzie should feel she must give this up. She is afraid of feeling deprived, but again, her perception plays a role. In digging through her family background, her mother never allowed ice-cream in the house. It was designated as a treat, but because Suzie was a heavy child, her mother would not give her ice-cream money. Now, Suzie gravitates towards ice-cream. She perceives it as a wonderful but sinful treat. If she perceived the world differently, she would see ice-cream merely as a dessert. There would be no emotion attached to the experience at all, and then she would be able to take it or leave it.

Finally, Suzie's third objection to starting a weight loss program is attached to the notion that everyone will be watching her. This is a fear that is not as simple to resolve as the other two. The first fear discussed of not being able to eat wedding cake, and the second of not being able to indulge in ice-cream, are easily ameliorated. However, the idea that people will be watching her progress is more complicated. This objection relates to a deeper conflict. When she thinks about attempting to lose weight, she feels vulnerable. What if she fails? What if she receives criticism about the plan she selects? Discussing dieting can bring up some controversies and perhaps she does not want go there. She would rather avoid any uncomfortable discussions by ignoring the issue entirely and this can be accomplished by not losing weight. Even if Suzie diets without telling anyone, they will surely begin to notice as the pounds drop off. She will be forced to discuss her weight.

While Suzie's experience may be typical, it is not the only experience. Again, every woman brings her perception to the table. Not everyone feels the same way. Many people lose weight and they talk about it. In fact, many people are proud of their accomplishments. A good number of people who are upset about being overweight do not mind discussing the subject. Some people actually like to talk about diets and weight loss, no matter how big they are. Therefore, it is Suzie's perception that holds her back. It is her opinion that talking about dieting is to be avoided. Perhaps this point of view stems from her earlier years when her mother was always on diets and always talking about it. Suzie perceives weight loss as negative and made a decision years ago that she would not talk about it. She did not want to be like her mother.

Suzie's unique filter—her perception—would take in all of her sensory experiences, and her intuition, and come up with reasons why she could not successfully lose weight. Obviously, with so much negativity and a feeling that she could not succeed, it is likely that her intuition was turned down like a burner on a stove. If you imagine that a flame on the stove is your inner core, and you turn down that flame, you will hardly feel it, but if you turn it up—through meditation and through really listening to your intuition--you will begin to sense it. Turning the flame up is not particularly difficult.

As you delve more into the inner you, you will get in touch with who you are and your perception will change

Perception is merely a filter, much like a sieve. When you are born, you begin not with a tabula rasa or blank slate, but with tendencies dictated by your DNA and from your experiences that started in the womb. The baby girl is new and pure. She is open and ready to absorb information. The baby discerns between likes and dislikes and has simple emotions. She wails at something that disturbs her, and she smiles at something that gives her pleasure. The filter works by taking in every part of the human experience—the five senses of sight, sound, touch, taste, feel, and intuitive messages—and interpreting all of the information. Information in the environment encounters the filter before it is able to enter the mind. While the infant's filter is new, the aging process alters it, and this starts immediately. It is altered by how long her mother waits to pick her up when she cries, and it is altered down the road by her teachers and relatives. As she enters adulthood, her sieve with which she interprets the world is unique, and far from the one she started out with on her birthday, but it never stops changing. Over time, it may become dirty. Sometimes it becomes so clogged that it will not take in any new information, but other filters are more open. Some people keep them clean by exercising their minds, participating in new experiences, and allowing change. Change flexes the filter. Meditation washes the dirt away.

If someone has a clogged, dirty, or faulty filter, the input to the brain will be different than for someone who has one that is clean or completely open. An example is that someone hears of a new local political candidate. One person might be excited by the prospect of a new face in the political party with which she is affiliated. Another person, who might even be a member of the same party, is less enthusiastic, suggesting that all the candidates are the same anyway. The first individual has a filter that is more open than the second person that sees things rather cynically. It is not that one individual's perception is wrong, but if the sieve is clogged, the information cannot be processed by the mind. When you close your mind, you weed out information, and when you do that, you cannot let in new ideas. So when you hear of a diet regimen, and you are closed off to the idea due to your old experiences and beliefs about dieting, your perception may prevent it from coming in. However, if you change the way you think by getting in touch with the inner you, that will change. Your filter will be cleaner, and it will permit the flow of positive information. It is also important to realize that perception serves a purpose. Not all information is good, so there will be things you want to keep out, but having an open mind—or letting the ideas in—only allows us to entertain new thoughts. We always have the option of rejecting the ideas.

Each filter is unique because we all have different experiences. Your perception on some level is what makes you who you are, but if your filter is seemingly causing you to think negatively, or to be closed to opportunities, it is not serving you well. You never want to replace it completely as that is a part of you, but you might want to tweak it once in a while. It is certainly possible to clean the sieve. But take care not to scrub it hard. This implement is something that has been a part of you since birth and it needs attention, and tender loving care, but you do not want to give it an overhaul. So how do you gently clean your filter? Meditation and getting in touch with your self will make a tremendous difference, as will questioning your thoughts. Every time you create something new, question existing thoughts, or entertain the ideas of others, you are allowing things to change. When you decided you might be willing to try a new sport, or that you might want to attempt calorie counting again, you were exercising the muscle that helps to alter your perception. As time goes on, and if you are open to new ideas, you will change your mind. Your mind will be altered due to a change in your perception, and that makes all the difference in the weight loss process.

Notes

Part II
The Active Phase

CHAPTER 6

PLANNING AND GOAL SETTING:
PERSONALIZING THE PROGRAM

Welcome to your new life. It is a life filled with movement, good healthy food, and a sense of inner confidence. You are about to embark on a weight loss journey and the end result will be a new, slimmer you. Hopefully, you have read the first part of this book and you are ready to start the active phase of the program. Ideally, this book is read chronologically, but it is okay if you find yourself here prematurely. You are curious, and want to know what the plan will entail. Will you have to give up your favorite foods? Will you have to exercise? Will you feel deprived? The answers to those questions are no, yes, and hopefully not. However, if you have been searching for an eating plan that is not too strict, and one that will actually work, you have found the right book. There is nothing "strict" about this plan. In fact, you are ultimately the designer of your program. Suggestions are offered for those who prefer structure, but there is a great deal of flexibility. You will never feel limited when going out to dinner, or attending a wedding, or just selecting foods at the market. You will no longer fear having ruined your diet because you cheated. There is no such thing as cheating on the *Change Your Mind* program. There is no food police. There is only guidance and structure, but no real limitations. The only limitations you feel are those you impose on yourself. How can that be true? After all, you will be restricting the amount of food you eat, you will be exercising, and while this is not a lightweight read at all, some of you may be wondering how it is that these claims can be made. How is it that you can lose weight by changing your mind?

The answer is one that cannot be explained. It must be experienced. The importance of reading the first part of this book cannot be overemphasized. If you read Part I, you will understand why changing your mind changes everything, and how everything will click once you integrate the information. At some point, a level of trust develops, which is equated with the idea that you can do this if you read the book. And you will see that your new life will materialize if you give the method a chance.

Once you finish reading the first portion of this book, read this second part, but before you begin to implement the active phase, you have to know from where you are starting and where you want to go.

Where Are You Now?

You are testing the waters, you are learning who you are, and you are changing just a bit at a time, minute by minute. Life is not static. Everything changes all the time. The cells your body started out with this morning are different now. You breathe in the air that others breathe out, and what you breathe out goes into the universe and this process may be looked at as a natural way of recycling and a natural manner of connection. With the remarkable breath, we connect ourselves to everything around us, and while that may be obvious, what is not so obvious is that with every moment of your life, you are changing.

When you started this book, you were a different person than you are now. Of course, that is not entirely true. You are still you, but you have grown a bit emotionally, psychologically and spiritually, so there is a difference between where you are now and where you were when you first started to read this book. Similarly, other people who are reading the book are changing too, and they are different from you because each has a different life path, different goals, and different struggles, so it is important to personalize this plan and create unique goals. While you may have a goal in mind, it is important to understand where you are right now, and that starts with an assessment of the physical you.

Stepping on the Scale

This is much more than a weight loss book, but if you are reading this book, it is likely that a significant goal for you is to lose a certain number of pounds. You may want to lose 25 pounds or more, or you may want to lose only 5 or 10 pounds. Either way, in order to determine how much weight you want to lose, you have to start with your current weight. We know this is not something you want to face. You may have been avoiding the scale, but in order to begin the process, you have to know the truth. How much do you weigh?

Decide on which morning you will start the "weigh in" process. Then, on that day, before you even brush your teeth or drink a glass of water, step on the scale. Engage in this process monthly-not weekly, not never again-but once each month on any day of the month you like.

Record your weight here: _____.

By only weighing yourself monthly, there is ample time to see a drop in weight, and it is not too frequent where you will be witness to the meaningless but inevitable ups and downs. Each month, record your weight on the designated page in the coaching section, or in your notebook. Next, decide on a specific weight loss goal. Use your personal experience, body mass index (BMI), and body fat percentage to help you create a weight range goal. The first thing you need to do is to think about your personal history.

Your Personal Experiences

Think about a time when you were happy with the number on the scale. This will not necessarily be your goal weight because you are older now. Adolescence, pregnancy, perimenopause, and menopause are times when women experience enormous shifts in their bodies. In fact, there is hardly a decade that goes by that a woman does not witness a dramatic change in her appearance. This is a natural evolution. As you age, your body will change its shape, and this means you have to re-examine your weight goals many times in your life.

Keep in mind that the body is supposed to slow as you age. Your metabolism slows down, and you may put on a few pounds. It is logical. Think of the infant that grows at a rapid rate. Her body is constantly growing and changing its shape as she goes from entering the world as a newborn, to a crawling and climbing infant, to a toddler that can hardly sit still. As she becomes a child, her body changes again, and remains relatively constant until it grows into preadolescence, which takes her to the start of another drastic developmental transformation.

Think back to when you were ten or twelve, and then remember how much your body changed from that time until your final year in high school. If you remember being slim before graduation, your body was probably much different than it is today, and for good reason. Your body was not fully developed at that point. You were still growing even though you looked all grown up. Think about how your body has transitioned. Then think about how you want your body to look now. You likely have shed your desire to look like a teenager who is uncomfortable in her own skin and instead, you want to look like the strong, intelligent, healthy woman that you have become, just smaller. Like a sculptor carving from a solid rock, you can mentally chisel your way down to the beautiful body you were meant to have. To see yourself in your future body takes practice, but it is worth the effort.

The Body Mass Index

The BMI or body mass index is nothing more than comparing your height and weight. As you are losing weight, you should aim for a BMI of under 25 but not less than 18.5. Use the following formula to calculate your BMI:

<u>Your weight in pounds x 703</u>
Your height in inches x height in inches

For example, someone who is 5 feet tall and weighs 150 pounds, would perform the calculation this way:

$$\frac{150 \times 703 = 105450}{60 \times 60 = 3600} \quad = \quad \frac{105450}{3600} \quad = 29.3$$

Use the same formula, and record your BMI here _____.

According to the Centers for Disease Control, a BMI below 18.5 is underweight, but when the BMI is between 18.5 and 24.9, it is considered normal. Anything over 25 is either overweight or obese. The obese range starts at 30. If you like, calculate your BMI periodically and enter it after you record your weight on the chart located at the end of this chapter. You need not do this frequently, but it is motivating to see that your BMI will improve as you lose weight.

Know Your Body Fat Percentage

Go to a gym, a university, or a medical office in order to access an electronic body fat percentage analyzer. The reason why this is important is that your body fat percentage is a reflection of the balance between fat and muscle in your body. Because muscle is denser than fat, body weight is not always a reliable indicator of progress.

My body fat percentage is: _____.

The ideal body fat percentage depends on your age. The younger you are, the lower your body fat percentage should be. According to the American Council on Exercise (ACE), average women have between 25 and 31% body fat, but those who are physically fit can have a body fat percentage as low as 21% and still be healthy. Athletes will have body fat percentages that are even lower than that. Anything over 31% is considered unhealthy. This is another measurement that you will want to record periodically. It will indicate how much fat you are losing.

Determining Your Weight Loss Goal

Weighing yourself, evaluating your history, calculating BMI and discovering your body fat percentage, lays the groundwork for a proper start towards creating your weight loss goal. Your doctor will also have valuable input. Employing these methods will help you to understand that you need to look at the whole picture and not just one number that appears on a chart. You are unique, so embrace that and start from where you are. Know that whatever goal you set is nothing more than a number that is easily changed.

Also, it is important not to focus so much on the number that appears on the scale. Rather, consider how you feel. Some of you know exactly where you want to be. You may be clear about your goal because you know where you look and feel best. Others may not be so sure. You may set a goal, get there, and realize you want to lose another five pounds. Conversely, you may set a goal and halfway through realize you look fabulous and feel great. If the latter happens, you don't have to continue to lose weight. Keep in mind that as you work out, your body shape will change. You may not need to lose as much weight as you thought, but of course, you won't know until you start the process.

When determining your goal, you should come up with a range of pounds as opposed to a single figure. Refine the goal to a five-pound range. Perhaps you will fall between 125 and 130, or 130 and 135. By deciding on a weight range, you will better be able to meet your goals. Trying to keep your weight at one particular number is unrealistic. Bodies are always changing, and our weight fluctuates due to the amount of water we retain as well as other factors, so your goals should be similarly flexible. If for example you weigh 150 pounds, your BMI is 29, and your body fat percentage is 37 you would likely want to lose some weight. So you think back and realize that you were happiest when you weighed 130 pounds and wore a size 8 dress. You know that it would be reasonable to lose twenty pounds. You can even use your target weight and plug your numbers into the BMI formula to see what you get. Will your goal weight put you in a healthy BMI range? If so, it is probably a reasonable goal. When you determine a good weight, allow for small changes. Instead of saying you want to weigh 130 pounds, create a target weight range of between 128 and 133.

To begin, set a goal now, and start to see yourself as the person you will become once you lose the weight. After recording your weight, noting your BMI and body fat percentage, speaking with your doctor, and thinking about your past weight losses, if you have not come up with a range, just start with a small goal. Opt to lose five or ten pounds. Then, after you reach that goal, reassess the situation. Although you will be setting a goal, your body will shrink in its own time. On some level, your goals are just guidelines. If you follow the program, you will be losing weight at a healthy rate. Don't get hung up on how much weight you will lose each month. No matter what weight loss diets claim, you really don't know how much weight you will be able to lose until you start a program because everyone's body is unique. After you set a goal weight, you can track your progress through noticing how much room you have in your pants, by looking at yourself in the mirror, and by weighing yourself monthly. After examining the different concepts in this section, thinking about your personal situation, and giving this all some thought, let it sit for a while. In a day or two, come back to this section and write down your weight loss goal:

I want to weigh between _____ and _____.
  Today's Date:

Congratulations! You have set a goal and so you have taken the first step towards changing your life, and losing those excess pounds for good!

Weight Loss Goals Beyond the Scale

It is obvious that you bought this book because you wanted to lose weight, but what are your specific weight loss goals? You might have the goal of getting into a dress that has gotten too tight, or to be thin enough to fit in the crawl space of your basement, or to just be able to see your waist again. Some women have a tendency to think about tangible goals, but the best part of your weight loss is the feeling you will experience once you reach your desirable weight. There is no feeling like the feeling that arises when you achieve something for which you have been striving. You will feel good because it took courage to do it, and you will feel good when you get compliments on your weight loss, and you will—believe it or not—feel good when you are engaging in physical activity.

Now, think about what it will feel like to be slim and healthy. Your imagination will take you to a place where you are not only much thinner, but where you will be leading an active lifestyle. Imagine yourself getting up an hour earlier every day and going for a jog, and then coming home, taking a refreshing shower and enjoying your breakfast before you head off to work. You grab an apple to eat at your desk in a couple of hours, and that will keep you until lunch. Your co-worker walks by with doughnuts, eyeing the shiny apple on your desk, and while she offers you one, you do not feel guilty about saying no, nor do you even want the sugary round thing. You no longer have a craving for it. As she walks away, you wish that she would be healthy too as you bite into your apple. Later, you go to the clothing store during your lunch break and try on a pair of jeans. You realize that now you are a size smaller than you used to be. On the way back to the office, you stop at the deli and order a chicken wrap, eat it at your desk and feel fully satisfied with your healthy choice. This is an example of a mental movie, but yours can be anything. If you imagine you are there, you soon will be. That is the power of imagination.

Planning for Weight Loss

Planning to start a weight loss program is similar to the planning of a new career, or the development of a new hobby. For example, if you decide that you want to completely change careers, you would think about it. You would examine your career options and take the decision very seriously. You realize that enhancing your career will ultimately lead to satisfaction, greater self-esteem and a happier life. You would examine what you need in terms of education, how you would rearrange your schedule to accommodate any necessary instruction or training, and how it all fits into your schedule. You would also weigh your options. Say you are a clerk in a record store, and you want to become a doctor. That is a tremendous leap. However, you would not just suddenly quit your job and go to medical school. You would research the career to see if it is a good fit, and then you would assess your abilities. Do you have the education required to apply to medical school? If you decide that yes, you really want to become a physician and you meet the requirements, you would begin to prepare for the MCATs. Next, you would take the test, and apply to medical schools. When you are accepted to a medical school, you have to decide whether or not you can afford to quit your job at the record store, and how your finances will work during your stint in school. You may have to put your social life on hold because this level of education requires an inordinate amount of studying and training. You will experience a significant shift in your lifestyle and you have to understand that before you begin.

By comparison, losing weight seems easy, but the steps you take to accomplish the goal are exactly the same. First, you would ask yourself what you would gain when you lose weight, just as you did when you asked yourself what you would gain if you changed careers. Going from a store clerk to a physician would mean greater satisfaction. In contemplating the change, you would visualize the lifestyle. You might see yourself having dinner at a fancy restaurant and being interrupted by a pager. You excuse yourself to take a call, go outside, provide good advice to a patient, and then feel satisfaction as you head back to the table. You utter "false alarm," and go back to your steak dinner, smiling because your satisfying career provides you with a lifestyle you enjoy.

When you go from being sedentary and overeating to a lifestyle where you are slim and attractive, you might visualize your friends and family waving to you as you finish a triathlon. After you are done, you feel like a champion and you and your new running buddies go out to celebrate that evening. Both major changes lead to a significantly improved lifestyle. The "before" reality might be that as a record store clerk, you would go home and watch television after work, and feel unfulfilled. The "before" version of the weight loss vision might be that you also plop down on the couch and watch television. In some manner, no matter what type of positive change you make, your life will be remarkably better, and interestingly, any type of change requires the same steps. Changing careers—record store clerk to doctor—requires research, assessment, making the time necessary to accomplish the goal, and fitting it into your life. When you plan to lose weight, you should also think about the same things.

Like a career change, you will need education before you lose weight. Unlike pursuing a medical career, you need not go to school for years. In fact, this book provides all the education you need to learn how to lose weight. You also need an assessment. The material in this chapter helps you to examine where you are now and where you are going. Then, you choose a plan, and implement it, which means that you need to make the time for it in your life. If you were making a career change, you would automatically clear the way to have sufficient time to invest in education, training, and working. You would assess your life, evaluating whether the things you need to do fit with your current situation.

If you were to go to medical school, you might examine whether you will need after school care for your children, whether your car will make the trip to the school on a daily basis, and how you will handle mundane decisions like packing lunches, when the dog will go to the groomer, and when you will have time to do the weekly food shopping. All your ordinary activities must be considered and possibly rescheduled. You may need to rearrange childcare, or buy a better car, find a place to eat a packed sandwich, groom the dog at home to save money, and do the food shopping on Sunday nights with your children instead of right after work. Similarly, when you lose weight, you examine how exercise fits into the equation, how you will be shopping differently, and what you will need in order to reach your goals. What do you need in order to lose weight? You need this book, a notebook, a scale, some exercise equipment, and a visit to a gym to glean your body fat percentage. What is perhaps most important in preparing to lose weight is to clear enough time to exercise and meditate, which translates to only about an hour a day.

It is not difficult to fit an hour per day into your schedule but you have to decide in advance when you will engage in each activity. Otherwise, it is too easy to skip a training or meditation session. Will you get up each morning an hour earlier so you can exercise before you go to work, or will you do it in the evening? It doesn't matter when you exercise or meditate. The important thing is to decide in advance when you will do it. For meditation, you need to pick a quiet time. If you live with other people, this can be challenging. Similarly, exercise can be difficult to squeeze in if you have a demanding career. You will want to look at your schedule. Maybe you can get in a half hour of walking during your lunch hour, or you can take your kids to the park on Saturday while you run around the track. You might want to join a gym that is open twenty-four hours per day, or you might take advantage of gym equipment that your company offers. When choosing a quiet time to meditate, think about the rest of the family's schedules. If you live alone, think about outside noises like chatter from the neighbors who are sitting on the porch, or music that is being played too loudly in the evening. You might find morning the best time to meditate. Conversely, if the house is busy in the morning, you might prefer the slower energy that the evening usually brings.

Plan your meals and grocery shopping. Rather than trudging haphazardly through the market and grabbing what is on sale, make careful selections. Remember, you are making an effort to eat healthy, so you must be cognizant of what you plan to eat and then you must plan to purchase the correct ingredients in advance. Preparation will help you avoid having to make a fast food run because there is nothing appetizing in the house. Of course, if you find yourself at the drive-through window, know your options. Research nutrition facts for fast food restaurant meals even before you get in your car. Many fast food establishments offer salads and maybe one or two other healthy options. Still, you won't find yourself scrambling to find a tasty meal if you shop appropriately and perhaps prepare meals in advance. If you are cooking one meal, you may want to make two portions and freeze one. Whatever you decide, make a plan and stick to it.

When engaging in a weight loss program, there are other things to consider as well. For example, what will you do when your clothing gets too big? Will you hide the items in the back of the closet, donate them to Goodwill, or give them to a friend or relative? After all, you *will* be wearing different clothing in smaller sizes. That is a guarantee if you successfully lose weight. It is not a big problem, and in fact, it can be fun to think about the clothing styles you will wear after you reach your target weight. Still, you must plan for the change, and this is just an example of something that will change in your life. There are other situations that could arise for which you may be unprepared. That is why it is important to examine your goals and any obstacles you might encounter. The point is that the obstacles will not floor you if you plan effectively.

Planning so Obstacles Do Not Get in Your Way

You already know that you will face some obstacles. You might find yourself at a smorgasbord with fattening foods that you want to consume, or you may find that you skipped three workouts in a row and are wondering what is wrong with you. You may have eaten really well and lost weight, but you now find that you have plateaued. Do these issues sound familiar? These are some common thought processes, but the problem here is that these are not problems really. They are just negative thoughts. You look at fattening food and think that it is fattening rather than think about simply having a few bites of the coveted item to satisfy your craving. If you skipped a few workouts, so what! Instead of thinking you are deficient, think that you will begin to resume your exercise plan just like that. If the number on the scale doesn't budge, simply revisit the program, think about whether your goal weight is reasonable, tweak your calories, or add exercise. There are a number of things you can do to tackle any obstacle that gets in the way of achieving weight loss success.

It is good to know that you have options, but planning for these times can mean the difference between frustration and success. You need to know what you will do when these situations arise. As part of the exercises that follow, you will be listing circumstances that could derail you while you are in the throes of losing weight. Then, you will be thinking of ways to counteract the predicaments. For example, you may write that when you go to the movies you will be tempted to buy a bucket of hot buttered popcorn. What will you do instead? You might figure the calories for a small popcorn with no butter and order that. But then you think, you might feel deprived. Instead of the buttered popcorn, you might eat a portion of a chocolate bar so you still feel as if you are treating yourself, or you could share the buttered popcorn with a friend. If you choose to share, eat just two handfuls of the buttered popcorn and if you are counting calories, include them. Will you live the rest of your life feeling as if you want hot buttered popcorn every time you enter a movie theater? Absolutely not. As you embark on this journey, the foods that are calling you now will be completely irrelevant. You will not give them a second thought. But at the moment, these foods have power over you, so you have to deal with such situations by knowing where you are, anticipating what might happen, and figuring out how you will handle each and every one of these circumstances in the future.

If every time you start a diet, your husband brings home doughnuts just to tempt you, or your mother lectures you on what you could be doing better, you might want to respond to these situations differently. One way to approach them is to keep quiet. No one needs to know that you are counting calories in your head. No one needs to know that you purchased apples instead of apple pie because you are cutting calories. After all, this is a lifestyle change. You will grow to love the apples and not think about the apple pie, and while that seems unlikely perhaps at first, it is something that will happen. So when you stop buying junk food and replace it with healthy foods, it is a rather natural act. You do not have to explain yourself at all. Other obstacles might be when you are wrestling with inner demons. You might still find yourself, even after reading about how emotions affect you, plagued by cravings. How will you handle it this time? First, recognize that it is an obstacle, but again, there are solutions. Like you read in the popcorn example, you can eat a smaller portion, order popcorn without the butter, or eat a few pieces of a chocolate bar. Again, that is one example, but you can use the tools in this book to create solutions for your specific situation. When you encounter such an obstacle, you might want to re-read the chapter on emotions, and then go on to develop a pre-planned course of action.

Other obstacles may not be related to clothing or food. There are issues that are not weight-related but may cause you to veer off course. When you are losing weight, the rest of your life will contain many of the same elements. Things that would drive you to eat will still perhaps cause upset. Instead of running to the pantry whenever you have a disagreement with someone in your life, you may want to cultivate behaviors that will help you get through unpleasant feelings.

Meditation is a perfect tool to help alleviate stress, but there are other things you might want to do such as creating a list of rewards. Rewards could include buying yourself flowers, going to the movie theater or renting a DVD, getting a pedicure, or reading a chapter in a novel. There are many things you can do to replace undesirable behaviors with activities that you will enjoy much more. And while you may replace the negative behaviors with ones that feel better and will improve your life, it is important not to ignore persistent negative feelings. Such feelings indicate that something is awry, and exploring these feelings enhances self-knowledge, a result that will always bring you closer to achieving your goals. Carefully look at your life and decide whether you want to make changes, or at least delve more deeply into anything that is bothering you. You may want to address any troubling issues through psychotherapy or some other modality, but whatever you do, remember that nothing should stop you from losing weight. If you anticipate and plan for experiences that might have tripped you up in the past, weight loss will be simple.

When you find yourself eating for reasons beyond hunger, simply stop and assess the situation. Use the techniques provided in this book, or examine your life at your own pace and in your own way, and you will get through any difficulties. Above all, think of how you handle obstacles as an indicator of your personal growth. As you make your way through this life experience, you will handle things differently at different stages of your life. This is why you may lose weight this time, even if you have not done so in the past.

Planning and Goal Setting: Going Beyond the Weight Loss

By recording where you are now, planning where you will be, imagining your new self, and planning for obstacles, you are well on your way to the person you want to become. You may already have come up with a weight loss goal, but weight loss does not happen in a vacuum. It happens as part of your life. How do you see yourself in three months? What will your new skinny self be doing? You may imagine yourself doing all sorts of things that you avoided in the past. In fact, you probably want to make some changes--everybody does-- but don't wait to make those changes. So many people fall into the trap of putting off everything until they lose the weight, but your life goes on no matter what number appears on the scale. So think about the totality of your life, including your weight loss goals.

You may have always wanted to sing on stage but are shy about using your voice in front of an audience. If that is your dream, take baby steps. Take a singing lesson or join Toastmaster's-- the organization that helps people get over their fear of speaking in public--or just practice by singing in the shower. Perhaps you are a regular at the karaoke bar but have always been afraid to pursue a college degree. If that is your dream, go to the school you have been eyeing and browse the course catalog. Then talk to someone in the Admissions Department and find out what it would take to start on that path. In general, become comfortable with yourself. Losing weight might provide you with the confidence to finally pursue other goals, but again, losing weight is part of your life just as is honing a musical career or going back to school. Just do it, and do it all at once if you like. Do move at your own pace, but do not let fear hold you back.

It is important to think about what you want out of life. Although this is a weight loss book, the process of losing weight is again part of your whole life. It affects every aspect of it from the time you wake up until the time you go to bed. You make food decisions every day, and you also decide whether or not to exercise. If you are cramming activities into your day without leaving room for purposeful movement, you may end up not doing much exercise at all. Therefore, you have to think about your life as a whole. You have already begun to plan for exercise and that is a good thing, but you may have been holding back on your life because of your weight. When you lose weight, you may decide to make changes, and those changes may be uncomfortable or produce conflicts. It is precisely because of this that you ought to address these plans now.

Think of your life as it is, and think about what you want. Think about elements of your life such as your career, your relationships, your finances, and your soul needs, and create goals for each of these life areas. Many people do plan for changes in things that they feel matter, but they often neglect the most important elements. Soul needs are usually equated with passions or desires. Make sure to put these things high on the list of changes you want to make. Change your life now by making a decision to do more of the things you love, and eliminate some of the things that are not serving you well. You might choose to take an art class to explore your creative side, or you might decide to go skydiving just to experience the rush. You might want to adopt a dog, or you might want to volunteer at a shelter. There are many yearnings that lurk underneath your current life that could be fun to implement. By doing things you enjoy, you are making your life better. You will therefore be less inclined to use food as comfort because you will be involved in activities that enrich your life.

Use the following exercises to help you refine your weight loss goals as well as to establish your life goals. You may also want to create a precise plan to implement your life goals. Each week, simply look at three of your life goals. Ask yourself what one thing you can do during the week that will bring you closer to the goal, and do it.

It is important to realize that making other changes is not suggested merely to keep you busy and out of the kitchen, although that tends to happen when you are doing the things you love, as the point of all of this is to create the life you want. When you do things you love, you will likely forget about the time. You will be absorbed in the moment and be less inclined to overeat, or to eat out of boredom. Having a healthy, beautiful body is one part of your life, and you can achieve that goal by following this program, but the rest of it is up to you. The tools contained in this book are versatile. Use them for weight loss, but take them as far as you want. Change your mind. Change your weight. Change your life.

COACHING EXERCISES

Before you begin the active phase by starting a plan, purchase a notebook or if you prefer, use the space provided in this book in addition to the blank pages at the end of each chapter, and complete the written exercises. You might also decide to start a journal as that can be helpful as you experience changes.

Plan to take at least fifteen minutes each day of uninterrupted time to examine your goals and evaluate obstacles you might encounter. Examine all of your goals, and not just the ones pertaining to your physical body. If you don't have time to do that right now, that's okay. But plan to start the process sometime later today. Everybody has fifteen minutes. Perhaps you have some time before you go to bed, or maybe you have fifteen minutes after you are finished with dinner. Feel free to complete the exercises all at once or over the course of several days. Just go at your own pace. You may want to take time to reflect on the questions before you begin to write, but do what feels comfortable for you. When you complete the written exercises, you will have a helpful map to navigate your future. The exciting part is that you can incorporate these newfound goals into your life and your life will be that much more fulfilling.

Coaching Exercise 1: *What are your weight loss goals?* Remember, your goals are more than a number on the scale. It may be that you want to reach a certain goal weight, but you may have other weight loss goals related to clothing size, or losing a certain amount of inches around your waist, or being able to wear a clothing style that defines the new you. Make a list of all of your weight loss goals.

Coaching Exercise 2: *Brainstorm your life.* Sit down and write whatever life goals come into your head. What do you want out of life? What are your passions? What do you like to do that you do not engage in enough?

Coaching Exercise 3: *Make a mental movie of your new self.* You need not write anything down, but you may want to make notes. Choose a quiet space and time to lie down and close your eyes. Think about your weight loss goals, and your life goals. Then, while considering all of these things, make a mental movie of a typical day in your life three months from today. Don't only visualize. Feel it too. And integrate these visualizations and feelings into your consciousness on a daily basis.

Coaching Exercise 4: *Make sure that nothing gets in the way of your success.* What are the things or beliefs that have stopped you or derailed you in the past? How are you going to counteract each of these potential obstacles this time?

Coaching Exercise 5: *Create a Rewards List.* Simply think of things you will reward yourself with that are not food related. For example, you might reward yourself with a pedicure, a bubble bath, or a movie night.

Coaching Exercise 6: *Planning to Implement the Exercise Plan, the Nutrition Plan and a Meditation Practice.* Do read Chapter 11 first and come back to this page to answer the following questions:

1. When will I plan menus? When will I do the food shopping? When will I cook?

2. What types of aerobic exercise will I do?

3. Which days, and what time of the day, will I engage in exercise?

4. When and where will I meditate?

Weight Loss Record

Month	Weight	BMI	Body Fat Percentage	Comments

Notes

CHAPTER 7

THE PROCESS OF LOSING WEIGHT

You now know how your body works, and you also know that you are more than the sum of your body parts. You are more than your mind—the thinking part of you that is associated with the brain—because you accept your spiritual nature. You now may be aware of all this but while reveling in that knowledge is a good thing, there is also the danger of becoming complacent. That is, even if you know who you are, and you are making strides in your personal development and even your body composition, you must recognize that the journey you are on requires perseverance, patience and the understanding that weight loss is a process.

Why Weight Loss is a Process

What is a process? Why is it so important to understand the nature of weight loss in this way? That weight loss is a process is fundamental to understanding the nature of change. When we make changes, we like to think we are mulling things over, then making a decision, and finally, implementing the new condition. But this way of acting is often compromised by our own minds. What usually goes wrong is that we expect perfection so we give up even before we have begun to engage in the process. An example is that you decide to go back to school but just before you are ready to enroll, after having made the decision to forge ahead, the tuition bill arrives in the mail on the same day you learn that you need a new roof. You begin to second-guess the decision you so thoughtfully made, wondering if you really can afford to be doing this. You begin to feel selfish and foolish. While those thought forms dance in your head, you learn that your new boss expects you to put in more overtime. Although more money is certainly desirable, you worry that if you go back to school and put in a lot of work hours, you will not have much time to study. In this example, you make a decision and then you change your mind because of the way you are thinking about changes that are occurring in your environment. You may give up on the idea of going back to school. It never seems to work out for you anyway, you think. Of course, such a thought process is counterproductive. What you have done is to allow negative thinking to influence your decisions. The truth is that if you never pursue your dream of going back to school, it is not because of the external obstacles. It is because of the way you think. You have already learned that thoughts are very powerful. When you think about all of the things that can go wrong, and believe that school is just not in the cards, you have given up. Yet, if you recognize that everything is a process, you can still have the goal of going to school even if you are not able to do so immediately.

When it comes to weight loss, you may not be ready to count calories today, but that does not mean you won't be able to do so in the future. You simply have to acknowledge all of the possibilities and keep an open mind. If for example you feel that there are too many obstacles in the way of your weight loss success right now, it does not mean this will be the case down the road. In fact, if you integrate the messages to come from this book, your mindset will eventually change. And when you change your thinking, you will feel differently, and you will be able to change your weight.

Making the decision to lose weight is a process. The actual effort to lose weight is a process too. The implementation of a new diet or exercise program is never static. It is always changing. When you embark on a training program, it is undesirable to perform the same exercises over and over again. If you continue to do the same exercises for months on end, your body will become accustomed to the routine. In fact, you should be changing your exercise routine every few weeks. The same concept applies to counting calories. You may start on a calorie program when you weigh 197 pounds, but when you are down to 150 pounds, your caloric requirements change. This does not necessarily mean you will need to alter your calorie consumption because your metabolism will increase during the process of weight loss, but you will need to re-examine your caloric requirements. Clearly, change is a part of any weight loss program. Yet, the idea of process goes well beyond merely tweaking our diet and exercise regimens. It is also aligned with the fundamental nature of the human psyche.

When you begin to embark on a program such as the one described in this book, you are already in the throes of it. Either someone told you about this book, or you found it while scouring diet book recommendations, or you heard about it on television. Something prompted you to purchase or borrow this particular book. Before this book was even in your thoughts, the process began. You know that the process has begun because if you are reading this book now, you are in a state of readiness. Barring someone holding a gun to your head, and forcing you to read this material, you are doing so willingly. Yet, you may be entering this phase from various vantage points. You might have stopped dieting for a while, having given up on losing weight altogether, or you might be rebounding from a failed diet plan. Either way, the thought that weight loss is something you desire entered your mind at some point. You went from gaining weight and overeating to a time when you thought that perhaps you want to make a change. Your journey may be equated with many failed diet attempts, or perhaps you made the decision that you want to lose weight for the first time today. In either event, it took a process to get to that mindset.

We already talked about the idea that self-knowledge and the understanding of the workings of your body will fuel your motivation. Indeed, when you know yourself and you are fully present, you are attuned to what you like to eat and how you want to move your body. It helps to know what your body needs and wants. When you understand how your body works, you will be more motivated to take care of it. As you grow spiritually, something that increases your confidence and the belief in yourself, you will be even more motivated to take care of the physical encasement that takes you on your Earthly journey. And while this is quite a clear cause and effect experience, motivation theory helps you to better comprehend the experience.

We already talked about Maslow's well-known hierarchy of needs where it is theorized that human beings are motivated by self-preservation, at least at first, but when it comes to motivation, process theories allow us to further categorize the experience. There are a number of process theories of motivation of which the most popular is a paradigm developed by James O. Prochaska and colleagues call The Transtheoretical Model of Change. Based on this theory, there are several phases of change, from the time when you first have a glimpse of what you might like to do, to a phase where you are performing the tasks to achieve your goal, to a time when you are maintaining your success. In describing the process of change as we see it, we embrace these popular motivation models along with the idea that going within, and knowing yourself, is key to the transformation.

The Process of Weight Loss

Weight loss is a process that begins when you start to think about the concept. At this point, you are either neutral or negative about the matter. You may automatically react to criticism about your weight, and in fact eat more because you are out to prove that no one can tell you what to do. Yet, criticism is not something that easily rolls off your back, so you keep the criticism in your mind and it festers. You may entertain thoughts about losing weight, even though you will vehemently deny this to your friends and family. Notions of weight loss enter your consciousness when you watch a television infomercial about a diet supplement or a piece of exercise equipment. You may quickly flip by the television channel, not wanting to see something about this topic, but again, the seed is planted. This thought form is a part of you now.

You may never get past this point, but again, if you have read this far in the book, you are probably past it so we won't even consider such a state of being as a possibility now. This means that you are probably at a point where you are at least thinking about seriously taking steps to lose weight. You are now taking initiative— again, if no one is holding a gun to your head-- and you may go from a position of saying that weight loss is not in the equation to one where you are seriously considering the idea. You are still reluctant, and you may be skeptical, particularly if you have been on many diets in the past. Yet, your mind is beginning to open. The thoughts that you are now thinking are moving in a positive direction. You consider some possibilities. You weed out the negative from the positive and look at options. At this time, you are thinking to yourself that maybe you will give a weight loss program a try.

You think about weight loss programs for a while, and then a significant shift occurs where you go from saying that you might embark on the weight loss journey to a resounding affirmation that you will do it. This is an exciting time because you are fueled by positive emotions that result from your new outlook and commitment to a goal. You may have already purchased a new pair of sneakers, or started to discuss dieting with a trusted friend. You may have entered the local gym to inquire about membership. Certainly, when you are excited about making the change, you are checking the labels in the supermarket to see which foods are healthy, and which contain too much fat and sugar. You are struck by the fact that you probably gobbled a thousand calories in a sitting because some foods are that calorie dense. You are thrilled that you can easily save calories by following a nutrition plan and still feel satiated. You are preparing now, but you still retain your old habits. You are excited because you are thinking about your goals and are visualizing how good you will look in a bathing suit, but you may be doing this while still engaged in overeating behaviors. That is okay. You are still moving forward. By this point, some of you may have already begun to move toward healthier habits. You are preparing for change.

You soon realize that there is a difference between talking your game and actually doing something to implement your plan, and you begin to take steps to live the program. By this time, you are probably exercising. You are counting calories, or you are on a certain food plan, or you are at least gravitating toward healthy eating. You are doing it now. You feel good because you are embarking on a new path. You are also being true to your word. You revel in your successes, but you sometimes miss the mark. When you do eat something you feel you should have skipped, you may develop feelings of inadequacy, but it is important that you do not give up.

This is the part of the journey where understanding this process can help. When you do feel negative about the program, stop and think about the situation for a moment. You now know that you are at a point where you are doing something. You may for example be counting calories. This is good, but there will be setbacks. For example, you may have eaten two doughnuts for breakfast and you know you will not have enough calories to make it through the day without experiencing hunger. You think that maybe you should just give up the diet because it is too hard for you, but if you stop dieting, you are no longer engaged in this process. However, it is precisely because you may have thought about a diet as being "on" one, or "off" one, that you have given up in the past. Remember, you are never off or on anything. Rather, you live your life and you make food choices every hour of the day. If you had two doughnuts for breakfast, what does that have to do with your choice for lunch? You can continue your day, while making better choices. And as for the calories in the doughnuts, you will probably be surprised at how long it sustains you. It may be true that you will experience hunger earlier than usual if you skip lunch, but if you had an inordinate amount of fat and sugar in the morning, you may not be hungry at your usual lunch hour anyway. You may find that eating a few pieces of cheese and a handful of grapes are all you need to get you through until your next meal. In this situation, when you feel as if you are failing, your Monkey Mind takes over. It is the feeling of failure that prompts you to think about giving up. There is no reason to give up when you understand that these situations are just part of a process, and not the end of a diet.

You may have gone off diets in the past because they felt confining or because you were not losing enough weight. Just knowing that weight loss is a process can help because you realize that you are not being good or bad. You simply exist. You are moving toward your goal, but it is not a direct incremental process without dips or backslides. There is forward motion, but sometimes you take a step back, or you take a step off to the side. By definition, no process is perfect, and when you realize that perfection is not an option, you will realize that you can relax and just enjoy the process. You will at some point reach your goal weight and feel as if you have succeeded. However, when you implement a diet and exercise plan, and even after you reach your goal weight, you are not done. The process continues, ushering in the concept of maintenance, where you continue a conscious effort to stay on course. By this time, you have already integrated the program into your life, but it is important not to become complacent. You will continue not only to be conscious of the state of your body, but you will become conscious about the state of your life. Again, weight loss is only one part of your life. It is likely that you will want to make other changes while you lose and maintain weight.

Are You Ready to Lose Weight?

Where you are in the process matters. You may have already read the first part of this book and are thinking about losing weight. You may not feel completely ready to take the plunge but you are interested in the goal. This is good. It means you are taking a step forward. At the same time, integrate the idea that losing weight is a process. You are either thinking about losing weight, or preparing to lose weight, or have even started to implement weight loss strategies.

Whatever state you are in, it does not matter in regard to success. You will be successful. Wherever you are, think of this present moment as part of the process. It is not necessary to think that you have to reach a certain point of readiness to begin. Simply, start from where you are. You will always move forward.

Reading and integrating the first part of this book is part of the process. If you are not ready to start the program, rest assured that if you continue to think about losing weight, you will be ready eventually. There is no reason to rush the process and there is no way to know how long it will take to get to a point of readiness. Understand that experiencing weight loss as a process is necessary in order to achieve lasting results, so it does not matter where you are on the journey. By knowing where you stand, you are empowered. Only you know when you are ready to go to the next stage in your development. Only you know when you are really ready to begin each strategy.

What if you are not sure if you are ready to implement one of the plans in this book? Actually, you cannot make a mistake. If you choose a plan, and then you have a setback, it is part of the process. It is always a learning experience. If you feel like you might want to try one of the plans, just give it a try!

Taking a Step Backward to Go Forward

It is not fun to feel as if you are slipping, or to gain a few pounds, or to find that your clothes are tighter, or to realize that you didn't make it to the gym once in the past week, but to really move forward you have to accept that you will never adhere to your plan exactly. So when you have a setback, realize that you are doing what you are supposed to be doing. You are engaged in the process.

Think of setbacks as a sign of success, and not failure. You can never fail because tomorrow is another day. You can always recover from any setback at any time in your development. Yet, it is helpful to recover quickly. If you ate something with way too many calories earlier in the day, it need not send you on a binge. Realize that small mistakes are part of the process and move on.

If you eat too many calories, or consume too much junk food, you then have to use your cognitive abilities to think things through. There are tools to help you with the rough patches. An example is that if you are planning to go to a dinner party, you may think that you will feel restricted. You have, up until that point perhaps, been adhering to a meal plan. If you are counting calories, one strategy is to make sure that you do not go to the party hungry. Do have breakfast and lunch, but if the event is around dinnertime, save the rest of the calories so you can splurge. Choose mostly healthy foods, but do have a taste of anything you want. Estimate the calories the best you can based on your acquired knowledge. If you have a small amount of high caloric foods, you will probably be able to stick to the plan quite easily. Do have a good time and don't worry about whether or not you counted correctly. As you become accustomed to eating less food, you will naturally reduce your intake and it will be quite easy for you to eat within desirable calorie parameters.

If you are on Plan B where you are not counting or measuring your food, you might want to just take a break from the restrictions. Use the Pause Button technique, where you stop thinking about nutrition and just take a break from the program. On Plan B, you are eating healthfully, but when you go to a party, you are faced with an array of fattening fare as well as things you do not ordinarily encounter. Sometimes, you will have no idea whether or not something is healthy anyway. If there is a food you want to eat, go ahead and try it. Press the Pause Button, but as soon as the party ends, resume your program. And of course, only use the Pause Button occasionally. Obviously, if you use it several times a week, your weight loss effort could be compromised. Use your judgment. If you attend numerous parties and events, use this technique once in a while and you will not feel deprived. The rest of the time, stick to healthy eating.

Another difficulty that people encounter is when there is an unexpected event. Life may take a negative turn. A loved one may be in the hospital or stress at work takes a toll. You may have slipped into old eating habits because of the negative environment. How do you get back to the right way of thinking, and the right way of eating? Simply stop and assess the situation. What happened? What are you doing differently? Then re-read the first portion of this book. Remember, you are not starting over. You are not starting a diet because this is again not a diet. Do not think of yourself as having gone off your diet. Rather, think of this situation as part of the process. After all, it is. These slips are inevitable. Life happens. You have done a great job of integrating the program, but if you have gone astray, simply resume the program as soon as you recognize the indiscretion. Never think that you failed, because you haven't. If you understand that losing weight is a process, these situations will never bother you.

Another thing that sometimes derails weight loss efforts is eating in restaurants. No matter what, if you eat out infrequently, your calorie estimates or decisions are unlikely to slow down your progress. This is because it is one meal, once in a while. Still, overeating simply because you can is not wise. You will be better off eating what you like in small portions.

On Plan A, you will want to find out how many calories your

planned order contains, or you can estimate calorie content based on the tools provided in the Plan A chapter. If you are going to a chain restaurant, it may be easy for you to look up the calories online in advance. If not, try to examine the menu. There may be things on the menu that you ordinarily do not eat, so it might be wise to prepare by finding calorie counts beforehand. If you are on Plan B, it is easy to make healthy choices in restaurants. If for example, a dish comes with rice, you might ask if it can be substituted with a vegetable. Many restaurants will accommodate special requests. Salad is always a good option when you are unsure of the quality of the food, but make sure to request the dressing on the side. Knowledge about food is key to making wise choices, and while many restaurants promote their most fattening dishes, there are always suitable meals you can select. Once you understand which foods are healthiest, and have begun to live the lifestyle, you will have enough knowledge to not only order appropriate foods, but to make special requests in terms of how you'd like your meal prepared.

Another situation that many dieters encounter is when they are confronted by food pushers, or people who cajole them to eat. It might be a well-meaning grandmother who already thinks you are too thin, or someone with a weight problem who does not want to see anyone successfully lose pounds. Either way, if someone is trying to get you to eat something you do not want, it provides you with the opportunity to take a stand. At first, you may politely refuse. As you lose weight, your confidence will increase. If in the past you ended up eating things you did not want simply because someone was trying to get you to eat a particular food, being on this program has the benefit of increased self-esteem so it will be easier for you to say no. However, if you are intrigued by the particular food, have a bite, and estimate its caloric content if you are on Plan A. You can even put some of the food on your plate, but only eat a bite or two. No one will notice what you leave over and you will not have to confront the food pusher. In the past, someone may have sabotaged your diet effort by trying to get you to eat something fattening. You succumbed and perhaps fell off your diet, only to feel frustrated by your lack of resolve. But when you are not on a diet, and you are just going through the process of weight loss, you can have a taste of something formerly forbidden and feel good about your decision.

Another issue where you may need flexibility is associated with cravings. Yes, you have made some changes, or you try to eat in a healthy manner, but you have had overpowering cravings in the past. How can you eat healthfully and not be plagued by thoughts of visiting your favorite drive-through window or buying a candy bar? First, realize that this is not a diet. This is not a plan of deprivation. If you want a candy bar, have the candy bar. If you are on Plan A, simply count the indulgence in the total calories for the day. In fact, if you have been emotionally eating in conjunction with these cravings, Plan A may be the best choice for you. You will be taking a quiz to find out which is the most suitable plan for your personality type, but when dealing with cravings, implementing boundaries provides a viable solution. Move toward healthy eating, but do eat some of your favorite foods. As you move through the process, you will have a desire for the healthier fare anyway. Again, this is a process, so do not be discouraged if you find yourself enjoying salads while also thinking about the candy bar.

What is important is that you now know the relevance of the process. Understanding that weight loss is something that you do as part of a larger change is important. The coping strategies provided helps you deal with obstacles you encounter on either plan. In fact, while reading through them, you may have an inkling as to which plan you want to try. You already have some information about each of the plans, but to really help you examine the choice, take the quiz in the following chapter and find out which plan would be a better fit for you.

Notes

CHAPTER 8

WHAT TYPE OF DIETER ARE YOU?

This program is not a diet, but it still pays to look at your diet personality. This is because you probably have some dieting experience under your belt, and these experiences will help you select the plan best suited for you. But before you take this quiz, think about diets you have been on in the past. Did you count calories or carbs or fat grams? Did you lose weight on these regimens or did you end up sabotaging yourself? Although the *Change Your Mind* program is really not a diet, your diet personality makes a difference when choosing a plan.

There are two plans from which to select. Plan A provides the easiest and most effective type of food boundary which is calorie tracking. While a good choice, some people are resistant to counting calories perhaps due to negative experiences in the past, or due to a fear of limiting themselves. If in fact you are used to binge eating, or you are accustomed to eating whatever you want in whatever quantities you like, learning calorie counts, or restricting food intake may present challenges. Of course, on this plan, you are provided with new tools that allow for an effortless way to count calories. If in fact you resisted this method because of the tedious nature of the approach, you might be pleasantly surprised when you discover the tools and techniques provided in Plan A.

Plan A and Plan B do have elements of what many diets

include. That is, while not considered diets, both plans prompt you to implement dieting techniques. Plan A relies on the good old calories in/calories out formula. Once you determine approximately how many calories your body burns, use the chart to help you choose a specific calorie plan. Then, tools are provided to show you how to count calories painlessly, and eat your meals in such a way to assure that your physical hunger is always satisfied.

Plan B takes a different approach by allowing you to get in touch with your hunger and to focus solely on nutritious foods. Each plan in its own way provides boundaries so that you will lose weight, but each also contains a great deal of flexibility to allow for personal preference. You may use the answers from the following quiz to help you decide which plan to choose. However, whichever plan you choose, you always have the option of changing mid-stream. Because, once again, losing weight is a process. If you find that the selected plan is not a good fit, you can change at any time. Now, are you ready to take the quiz? Just answer each of the questions as either True or False.

QUIZ: What Type of Dieter Are You?

1. I have counted calories in the past, and I have never lost weight that way.

2. I have failed at dieting in the past. Somehow, even though I think I am doing everything right, I do not lose weight, but I really push the boundaries.

3. There have been times in my life when I lost weight naturally, such as when I was in love, or I was really motivated to lose weight for an event. I don't know how I did it. I guess I just ate less and it worked.

4. I tend to overeat when I am angry, or sad. I am definitely an emotional eater.

5. I do best on diets when I am counting something such as calories, carbs, or fat grams. Left to my own devices, I have never been successful at cutting down on food.

6. I have cravings that seem overwhelming at times. I don't want to give up my favorite foods.

7. I really don't have much weight to lose. I have been successful in the past, and I have maintained my weight for a long time, but I just can't lose those last 10 pounds.

8. My diet is already focused on healthy food. I don't know why I am not losing weight. I guess I just eat too much of it.

9. I have never dieted before but I am willing to try anything.

10. I am a free spirit. I don't like rules. Just send me on the path and I will embrace the lessons I am given.

Scoring: If you answered TRUE to questions 2, 4, 5, 6 and 9, score one point each for Plan A. If you answered TRUE to questions 1, 3, 7, 8 and 10, score one point each for Plan B. Use the following guide to help calculate your score:

1. If TRUE , score 1 point for Plan B.
2. If TRUE , score 1 point for Plan A.
3. If TRUE , score 1 point for Plan B.
4. If TRUE , score 1 point for Plan A.
5. If TRUE , score 1 point for Plan A.
6. If TRUE , score 1 point for Plan A.
7. If TRUE , score 1 point for Plan B.
8. If TRUE , score 1 point for Plan B.
9. If TRUE , score 1 point for Plan A.
10. If TRUE , score 1 point for Plan B.

Interpreting Your Score: Simply choose the plan for which you have the most points. If you have a tie score, just start the plan that appeals to you. If you are uncertain, choose Plan A. Plan A provides the assurance that you are consuming fewer calories than you are burning. No matter which plan you think you want to try, read both the Plan A and Plan B chapters. There is information in both sections that is good to know, and also, you may reconsider your choice after evaluating each plan.

Notes

CHAPTER 9

PLAN A

Plan A, the calorie-based plan and the preferred method, is quite simple. You count calories. This is a rather basic method of losing weight. Yet, in the past, you might have found estimating calories difficult, or remembering how many calories you consumed, tedious. You might have given up calorie regimens because by the time dinner rolled around, you were already out of calories. Some of your past attempts at calorie counting might have been thwarted because you never allowed yourself enough calories, or you ate too many calories of the wrong foods. It could be that you were tripped up by understating calories in foods, and this caused you to put on weight. At those times, perhaps you felt as though you were fooling yourself and no matter what you did, you would never lose weight. You concluded that calorie counting does not work for you. If you have been unsuccessful at calorie counting in the past, don't worry. This calorie counting plan is easy. All the work is done for you. All you do is follow the rules. And if you don't like rules, that is okay too. You can break them and still remain on the plan by implementing alterations to suit your lifestyle.

The suggested exercise program contained in Chapter 11 begins slowly, but if you follow the regimen, you will be exercising six days each week so you can consider yourself moderately active throughout the course of the program. The caloric intake is estimated based on the assumption that you are following the exercise plan or something equivalent. Although being sedentary is really not an option on this program, it is possible for those who cannot exercise for medical reasons to implement the eating regimen. If that is the case for you, consult a medical professional to discern a proper calorie level and then just follow the plan. Similarly, if you weigh more than 200 pounds, a personalized recommendation is appropriate.

You already know how much you weigh. With that information, and a commitment to moderate exercise, look at the chart below to discover your calorie recommendation:

If you weigh	Choose
144 lbs. or less	1200 calorie plan
Between 145 and 179	1500 calorie plan
Between 180 and 199	1800 calorie plan
200 lbs. or more	2100 calorie plan

Next, select your plan based on the criteria above:

1200 Calorie Plan: Eat four 300 calorie meals.

1500 Calorie Plan: Eat five 300 calorie meals.

1800 Calorie Plan: Eat six 300 calorie meals.

2100 Calorie Plan: Eat five 400 calorie meals plus a 100 calorie snack.

Although eating between 1800 and 2100 calories might prompt a substantial drop in weight even for someone who weighs more than 100 pounds over the norm, weight loss should be gradual to be healthy. Therefore, a woman who is significantly overweight should receive specific guidance from a medical professional that can tailor calorie and exercise requirements to her specific situation. Also, while the recommendations will work for most readers, choose a plan based on your personal experience. If you initially select a level based on the chart but find you are losing weight too quickly, or not quickly enough, take the plan up or down one notch accordingly. Every body is different. This is not an exact science. Along the same lines, when selecting a specific calorie plan, keep in mind that all you ever need to do is choose a starting calorie level based on your current weight. You will probably lose one or two pounds per week on this plan, but as you lose weight, you may not have to alter the amount of calories you consume. Your body will become more efficient at burning calories throughout the weight loss process so there may be no need to change it. Again, your experience should be your guide.

Once you are aware of your body's caloric requirements, and are ready to start, review the following chart with calorie meal recommendations. There are four plans consisting of 300 or 400 calorie meals. You can eat anything you want within that calorie range, but the consumption of healthy food is highly recommended. Also, it is important to space your meals as evenly as possible throughout the day to avoid hunger. Guidance for choosing foods wisely is contained in Chapter 11. You will also find meal suggestions in the following pages.

To make the transition even easier, prepare a personalized food list. Use your notebook or the page at the end of this chapter to record your favorite foods. Then, look up 100-calorie portions of each of the foods. An example of this exercise is as follows:

100-Calorie Food List

Food	Portion
Bologna	one thin slice
Chef Boy Ardee Cheesy Burger Ravioli	1/3 cup
Campbell's New England Clam Chowder	½ cup
Corn Chex	one cup
Spaghetti	½ cup
McDonald's fries	½ small order
Banana	one small
Cantaloupe	½ medium size melon

The list above is just an example of what you will be doing on a much larger scale. Just think of the foods you eat now, the foods you crave, and the foods you want to eat to improve your life. When you make a list similar to the one above, you can create meals. For example, you might have a cup of Corn Chex and a quarter of a cantaloupe for breakfast. The Corn Chex is 100 calories and the cantaloupe is half of what appears on the 100-calorie list, and is equivalent to 50 calories, so the total is now 150. Add about a half cup of skim milk to the cereal and your breakfast is now about 185 calories. You might add a hard boiled egg at 80 calories and a cup of coffee with milk, which takes you close to the 300 calorie level. By creating lists, and remembering the counts of calories in the foods you ordinarily eat, putting meals together is easy.

Counting Calories

Now you have figured out how many calories you need to eat each day to lose weight, and you have guidelines for when you should eat your meals. While flexible in that you need not stick to the recommended calorie counts per meal, eating at least 300 calories at a sitting will ensure that you do not get hungry before your next meal, as long as you eat nutritiously. After you read the chapter on nutrition, exercise and meditation, you will discover which foods will help to keep you satiated the longest. Another important thing is to keep it flexible. There will be times when 300 calories will not be sufficient, such as when you are going out to dinner or to a party. It is fine to save calories on occasion. For example, if you know you will be eating a larger dinner, you may combine two meals. An example of this is if you are on the 1800 calorie plan, you may want to eat a 300 calorie breakfast, a 300 calorie lunch and then, just have a 100 calorie snack, leaving 200 calories from that meal to go towards dinner. Dinner may be a combination of two meals or 600 calories, plus the 200, leaving you with 800 calories for the outing. Even after all that, you still have an additional 300 calories you can use for an after dinner drink, dessert, or a snack before bedtime. This is just an example of how you might want to alter the plan. The plan is flexible and should mesh with your individual lifestyle. For example, if you only want 200 calories for breakfast, don't force yourself to eat 300 or 400 calories. Save the calories for later. Ideally, however you decide to allot your calories, it is best to distribute them rather evenly throughout the day. Yet, there are occasions where you will be best off saving your calories for a special event.

The beauty of this program is that if you do eat the recommended number of meals, you will not have to remember how many calories you consumed by a certain point in the day. You just have to remember how many meals you have left. For example, it may be three o'clock in the afternoon and you consumed three meals. If you are on a plan where you are consuming 300 calorie meals, you have ingested 900 calories, but you don't even have to think about the calorie count at all. Think meals as opposed to calories. If you are on the 1500 calorie plan, you know you will still be able to eat a 300 calorie meal at 5 o'clock and another meal at perhaps 8 o'clock. Remembering meals consumed is easier than remembering calories. While the meal counting method makes things easy, you will have to hone your calorie knowledge.

One way of acquiring this knowledge is to use a calorie guidebook. Another way is to read labels. Packaged foods contain calorie information. Just be sure to read how many servings are in the container or you may end up eating twice as many calories as you think you are consuming. While produce stickers do not contain calorie information, calories for fruit and vegetables are easy to obtain from nutrition guidebooks or on the Internet. In fact, there are many ways to discern the caloric content of the foods you eat. One trick to counting calories painlessly includes a method of estimation simply through the use of your hands, a technique that is associated with portion control.

Understanding portions is key to effective counting. Even if you know how many calories are in a serving of filet mignon, if you do not know whether you are eating one or two portions, it becomes difficult to know how many calories the steak contains. Therefore, you need a quick and easy method of guessing how many calories are in a food item and again, the answer is in your hands.

A handful of anything is a good measure for a 100-calorie portion, unless it is calorie dense, such as a very rich piece of cheesecake. Your fist might be the size of an apple or a cup of fruit or a slice of bread. If you cup your hand, you will be measuring a 100-calorie portion of cereal. Don't become too concerned about vegetables. In fact, you can have as many veggies as you like without counting, with the exception of corn and potatoes, because most vegetables are very low in calories. Protein may be measured in a similar manner. Just one egg fits inside your hand, and the portion of a flat chicken breast that is the size of your palm may be about 100 calories as well. One small fast food burger patty also fits nicely in the palm of your hand. The patty alone is actually about 90 calories. But what about the filet mignon you can't wait to eat? If it were as small as a fast food patty, it would be the same count, but filet mignon is much thicker. Still, a 3 oz. portion of filet mignon is generally about 150 calories, so had you erred, you would not have been off by much. The steak contains more than 100 calories despite its size due to fat content. This is an important consideration. That 100 calorie portion may double if there is a heavy fat content. For example, a fatty piece of meat that fits in the palm of your hand can be 200 calories or more. Of course, calorie estimation is a learning process and it takes some time to develop the skill.

Other tips can help you make better estimates. If you find yourself eating something that is swimming in gravy, sauce or dressing, add an additional 150 calories. Of course, you can limit sauces and dressing by using less of it, or making a request in a restaurant to have it served on the side, and then reduce the calories accordingly. These are just guidelines. As you begin to learn the calorie counts of your favorite foods, you will come up with your own methods of estimation. Estimation should be used when you are eating in a restaurant or someone's home and have no resources to figure the count. As you begin to learn about specific caloric contents, you will retain some of the information, and calorie estimation will become much easier.

It is fine to estimate calories throughout the day, especially when you are out and cannot get exact figures. While this is acceptable, and will yield good results, use actual measurements and exact calorie counts when possible. This way, you will be assured that at least most of the time, your count is accurate. Although you probably will not go wrong while estimating healthy foods, when you are at a restaurant trying to figure how many calories are in a sliver of chocolate cake, you could run into trouble. Many restaurants serve calorie laden foods, and dessert is especially dangerous. Of course, if you are generally eating healthy and only go out occasionally, you do not have to be concerned about underestimating calories once in a while. However, if you are eating out a lot, and really are not sure of how many calories you are consuming, you might want to ask the wait staff or restaurant owner how a dish is prepared, and figure out how many calories you are really eating. Many chain restaurants post their menus with nutritional information online, and if you are eating at a fast food establishment, it is easy to find calorie counts. If you do not know the calories in the cake you are eating, figure about 400 calories for an average size piece. Obviously, you may decide to eat half, a strategy that will see the calorie expenditure at only 200, which is much more reasonable.

When you know what you will be ordering in advance, it is easier to properly estimate the count, but it is certainly not necessary to always know what you will be eating. After all, life is about adventure and you do not want to be the one who limits restaurant choices for a group simply because you are afraid of what might be served. Fear not. After you become better acquainted with calorie counts in general, you will get a feel for the technique of estimation and it will become second nature. Until then, it is okay if you stumble. There will be times when you eat a food that is very unhealthy and was probably more calories than you thought, but that's okay. Losing weight is a process, and you will reach your goal weight eventually.

Keeping track of calories is sometimes arduous. You can jot down the number or put it into a handheld device, but again, an easy way to count calories is to do it by meals. For example, the 1200-calorie plan allows for four 300-calorie meals. When you eat 300 calories for breakfast, all you have to do is think about your next meal. If you stick with the 300-calorie schedule, you need not remember how many calories you had throughout the day. All you need to do is remember how many meals you consumed.

You can eat anything you want at your meals. However, you will want to make sure you get adequate amounts of protein and include a variety of fruits and vegetables. The chapter that covers nutrition will help you to select foods that are best for you. The next few pages provide some suggestions for creating meals that are equivalent to 300 or 400 calories, and a 100-calorie snack list is also included.

300-Calorie Meals
BREAKFAST

❖ Two-egg veggie omelet, ¼ large cantaloupe wedge, one cup sweetened almond milk

❖ ½ bagel, low fat Laughing Cow cheese wedge, one cup orange juice

❖ One cup oatmeal, ½ c blueberries, one cup dark chocolate Pure Almond Milk

❖ One cup Wheat Chex, ½ c 2% milk, ½ c grapes, ½ c Greek yogurt, coffee with Half and Half

❖ One cup yogurt, one cup fruit salad, one hard boiled egg

LUNCH OR DINNER

❖ Turkey sandwich (six slices of thin-sliced turkey on 100 calorie whole grain sandwich round, lettuce, tomatoes, one tablespoon reduced fat mayonnaise), eight potato chips

❖ Big green salad with three ounces cooked chicken, two tablespoons croutons, one hard boiled egg cut in quarters, and one tablespoon reduced fat Cesar dressing

❖ Turkey burger (no bun), ½ cup green beans, ½ cup mashed potatoes

❖ One fast food hamburger (with bun), side salad with low calorie dressing

❖ One cup chicken noodle soup, baked chicken breast, cooked mixed vegetables

400-Calorie Meals

BREAKFAST

❖ Three-egg veggie omelet, ¼ large cantaloupe wedge, one cup sweetened almond milk

❖ One whole wheat bagel, low fat Laughing Cow cheese wedge, one apple, 1/2 cup orange juice

❖ Three four- inch blueberry pancakes, 1/8 cup pure maple syrup, one cup skim milk

❖ One cup Corn Chex, ½ cup 2% milk, one large apple, one serving Greek yogurt, coffee with Half and Half

❖ One Starbucks Vanilla Bean Frappuccino Blended Beverage, one Special K cereal bar

LUNCH OR DINNER

❖ ½ turkey wrap, unsweetened iced tea, one peach

❖ Big salad with 3 ounces cooked chicken, two tablespoons croutons, one hard boiled egg cut in quarters, and two tablespoons Caesar dressing

❖ Turkey burger on a bun, 20 sweet potato fries

❖ One Burger King Whopper Jr., diet soda

❖ Baked chicken breast, baked potato with small amounts of butter and sour cream, cooked mixed vegetables

100-calorie snacks

❖ Kashi Blackberry Graham soft baked cereal bar
❖ One banana
❖ Blue Bunny 100 calorie Butter Pecan Ice Cream Bar
❖ ¼ c hummus with raw vegetables
❖ One large apple
❖ 18 fat free Rold Gold pretzels
❖ Five Hershey's Air Delights Kisses
❖ 15 whole cashew nuts
❖ One cup Rice Chex
❖ 18 Cheez-It crackers
❖ 35 Honey Mini Teddy Grahams
❖ Four chocolate Pizzelle cookies
❖ One Nonni's biscotti, any variety
❖ Six graham crackers (1-1/2 sheets)
❖ 100 calorie bag of microwave popcorn
❖ ½ cantaloupe wedge
❖ One mozzarella cheese stick
❖ 14 raw almonds
❖ One medium sized pear
❖ One hard boiled egg

The suggestions contained in the last few pages will help you to see the possibilities. Yet, these are just examples, as is the admonition that every meal should be either 300 or 400 calories. Yes, this method will provide you with satisfying meals that will help you to navigate a new way of eating, but it is not essential that you divide your calories in the suggested manner. As long as your caloric intake is equivalent to the total for the selected plan, you're fine. The 300 and 400 calorie system will however give you a great deal of satisfaction because it will keep you satiated throughout the day. However, it is also a good idea to vary the plan based on your lifestyle, and so you might alter things a bit dependent on your activities. Simply use the eating plan as a guide to create your meals.

Some of you may wonder if you will be hungry if you only ingest 300 calories at a sitting. The answer is, probably not. It is very possible to eat full, satisfying meals that are equivalent to 300 calories, even if you are used to eating a lot more. This is because when you eat a number of small meals, your body is satisfied. You are not overworking your system by digesting large amounts of food. You will be hungry sooner, but that is okay. Because you are planning to eat four to six meals per day, you will not go hungry. You will probably be eating every three hours on most days. This is the plan that will work for the majority of readers because it provides appropriate guidance for healthy eating as well as parameters for portion control.

Although the calorie counting approach will give you the boundaries you need to create a lifestyle of healthy eating, there is another method. For those of you who feel as if you want to try a more flexible approach to eating, and believe you have integrated the psychological and spiritual aspects of this program, Plan B is for you.

Summary

❖ Choose a calorie level and discern your meal plan so that you know how many calories you will eat each day.

❖ Write a list of favorite foods, as well as healthy foods you plan to incorporate into your diet, and determine the size of a 100 calorie portion of each food. Use this list to create meals.

❖ Try to space your meals evenly throughout the day, which translates to about every three hours, but be flexible.

❖ Count calories with the help of calorie guides, labels and ` estimation. Remember, a handful of most food items is about 100 calories.

❖ Have the goal of eating nutritionally, or as close to nature as possible, but realize that weight loss is a process and you will be altering your eating habits at your own pace. Read Chapter 11 for more guidance.

❖ Feel free to have unlimited quantities of low calorie vegetables without having to count those calories.

❖ Remember, counting meals is easier than counting calories.

❖ This plan is part of a larger program of nutrition, exercise and meditation. In addition to eating a certain way, you will be engaging in purposeful movement and meditation on most days.

Notes

CHAPTER 10

PLAN B

Plan B is the alternate plan. The term "Plan B" is often used when a first attempt at anything is unsuccessful. People will ask, what is your Plan B if things don't work out? In this program, Plan B is really just another choice. It is not any less prudent to choose this plan than to choose Plan A. That said, the majority of readers will do better on Plan A. Plan A has a greater number of parameters that makes compliance more likely. At the same time, Plan B will appeal to those who do not like calorie restricted regimens and who eat in a healthy manner anyway.

If you choose Plan A, you will eat a set number of meals. The same strategy is a part of Plan B. Eat between four and six small meals each day, eat in a healthful manner as outlined in Chapter 11, meditate, and exercise. That is Plan B in a nutshell. Of course, there are a few things you should consider. If you have been overeating and gaining weight on three meals a day, you may wonder how you will lose weight if you eat twice as many meals. It is important to remember that you will not be overeating, and you will be eating healthy fare, and you will be doing some other things that will be explained as you read this chapter, and these things will help you stay on track. Again, you will read Chapter 11 before you implement this plan. Chapter 11 covers nutrition and exercise, but there are a few other considerations that will help you lose weight, and you will find those suggestions here along with information on key components of nutrition.

The essential things to remember are to get in touch with your hunger and fullness levels, include variety in your choices, consume largely healthy foods, control your portions, and eat regular meals. These suggestions may appear superfluous, but they are important, and it may take an adjustment. If you already read the first part of this book, then you know that this program is not a diet, but a way of life. If you are excited about eating good, healthy foods, and are committed to exercise and meditation, you will have little trouble integrating these suggestions into your routine. To use this plan successfully, you cannot align yourself with the diet mentality at all. For example, if you are not hungry and you already ate three meals, do not eat just because you are allowed more meals. That attitude is equated with the idea that you want to get all the food that is coming to you, but that is not an attitude conducive to change. It is an attitude that is associated with getting away with something. That kind of thinking does not put the health of your body first.

If you catch yourself waiting for the hunger, and really wanting to be hungry so you can eat again, then you have not gotten past emotional eating. You still want to eat even though you are not hungry. If you are still engaging in emotional eating, you may also be eating the wrong foods. In fact, if you have a hard time eating only healthy foods, it may be the case that Plan A will work better for you. Even if you think you want to plunge head first into healthy eating, you may not be ready to give up the cookies just yet. Although you will be eating healthy foods on Plan A too, there is more room for play food there. On Plan B, because you are not counting calories, even minor indulgences put you in danger of eating too many high calorie foods. For instance, you will not lose weight if you eat apple pie for dessert every night. You may be able to eat pie and not overeat, and feel good about it, but there are frankly too many calories contained in a slice of pie for it to be a reasonable daily food choice. This is true even if you bake the apple pie yourself and use largely nutritional ingredients. Eating a piece of pie on a rare occasion never hurt anyone, but you cannot eat high caloric, sugary foods on a daily basis and still lose weight. If, on the other hand, you have gotten past your cravings and in fact can easily wait to eat your meals, you are probably a good candidate for Plan B. When making your decision, take these things into account along with your quiz score from Chapter 8.

If you are reading this because you have chosen Plan B, go ahead and start. If you feel any discomfort, or feel as if this will never work, choose Plan A. For those who are Plan-B ready, this will be a satisfying shift from your present experience with food. You will embark on a new way of thinking about food, and you will understand that food is the stuff that makes your body work optimally so you will desire adequate nourishment. You will therefore choose delicious foods, and you will always listen to your body's signals.

Pay Attention to Your Hunger and Fullness Levels

Eat only when you are hungry and do not eat to fullness. If you have been overeating, knowing when you are hungry and when it is time to stop eating can be challenging. After all, if you do not wait for hunger to eat, it is not easy to know when to stop. What you can do to become acquainted with this concept is to start the learning process on a day when your schedule is flexible. On that day, wake up and have a small breakfast. Then, wait for lunch until you eat next. Notice if you are hungry in between breakfast and lunch. If you had breakfast at 7 or 8 a.m. you may be ravenous by noon. In that case, you could have a mid-morning snack such as a piece of fruit. Eating when you are hungry—as long as you eat healthy food and do not overeat—will not be detrimental. Remember, this is not a one-size-fits-all approach. Everybody is different. Someone may not be very hungry early in the day. If you are not very hungry even when noon rolls around, wait until you are. Eat lunch at 2 or 3 p.m. if that is when you first get hungry again. If you are eating healthy, and eating enough protein, fiber, and good fats, then your system will work well. You will eat to a point before you might feel full, and then you will get hungry again when your body needs more fuel.

Stopping your meal before you are full takes practice. At the beginning, just notice how you feel. Did you feel full after your last meal? If so, eat slightly less next time. Once you are eating healthy foods, eating when you are hungry, and stopping before you are full, you will begin to enjoy your meals more and eating will feel very natural. You may find that you become hungry more frequently. This is good. It probably means that you are eating less at your meals and not eating past fullness. You should eat to a point when you are no longer hungry and feel satisfied. This is the natural way to eat. As human beings, we are designed to use food efficiently. When we provide healthy food for our bodies, they work for us and not against us.

Eat a Variety of Foods

You've heard it before: eat a variety of foods. It is logical. If you eat different types of foods, you will end up with a variety of nutrients. Even if you never did this intentionally, your body has an inner knowing. It knows what is good for it. Theoretically, if you tap into your intuition, you would choose the right foods for your body every time. In the end, you would be eating in a balanced way. You would naturally eat a variety of foods. Who wants to eat the same things over and over again? But some of us do. We get into a habit of eating certain things, and while some of those foods may be perfectly healthy, the more different types of foods you consume, the more opportunities you have for experiencing different textures, different tastes, and different natural elements that are essential for the functioning of your body.

Again, your body has an inner wisdom about this, but the truth is that there are so many external triggers for eating today that it seems prudent to look at the recommended daily allowances for the various food groups. In other words, we tend not to listen to our bodies because we are faced with a barrage of television commercials, well lit fast food restaurants along the ride home from work, and dinner companions who have their own peculiar eating habits. On this plan, you will be listening to your body to see if it is hungry, and you will ask it what it wants to eat. Even so, it is prudent to use some sort of guideline so that you are eating in a balanced fashion. This way, you will be sure that your nutrition is at least adequate.

Recommended daily allowances vary over time. Many of you are probably familiar with the food pyramid that was promoted by the American government, but in 2011, the pyramid was replaced by the food plate. The food plate concept has been implemented by a number of nutritionists throughout the years, but with varying degrees of commonalities. In general, if you simply fill half of your plate with fruits and vegetables, a quarter with protein and a quarter with starch, you will be eating balanced meals. This is a reasonable method of assuring that you are eating well and it is consistent with most special dietary requirements. If you are a vegetarian, or you are cutting back on carbohydrates, this approach is excellent because vegetables are emphasized. If you are filling your dinner plate, simply fill half of it with veggies, one quarter of it with a starch such as a half of a baked potato, brown rice, or corn, and then fill the remaining quarter with protein. A three-ounce portion of lean beef or chicken, or a half cup serving of tofu, is ideal to complete the plate. Breakfast may be eaten the same way. Rather than consume half your meals in vegetables, consume half of your breakfast in fruit. You might have a half of a cantaloupe with cottage cheese and a slice of toast with a fruit spread. The next day, you might add strawberries and blueberries to your cereal and also have scrambled eggs. The day after that, you might choose half a bagel with a slice of cheese, pineapple rings, fresh squeezed orange juice and coffee. You have many choices. Simply eat in a balanced way by utilizing the food plate concept and consuming different foods every day.

Eat Only Healthy Foods

Eat as close to nature as possible, watch your intake of fat and sugar, and be cognizant of the quality of the food you are eating. That is a summary of the nutrition plan contained in Chapter 11. It seems like a tall order, but again, you will want to eat healthfully when you are ready. Think nutritious. You may take a handful of nuts, a small piece of cheese and an apple, and that could be one of your meals. Nuts are packed with the oils your body craves, but they have a high calorie content. If you sit down to have a meal, and you are eating nuts as a part of that meal, take just a handful and don't go back for seconds. Similarly, a small piece of cheese can be a part of a meal, but four 80 calorie cheese sticks is overkill. Fruits and vegetables are ideal snacks as well, and are generally low in calories and high in fiber, so they will keep you satiated. A good tip is to keep a bowl of fruit in the kitchen, something that will provide you with an array of nutritional food choices throughout the day. Also, keep raw vegetables in the refrigerator cut up for quick snacks. This can be very helpful too. Raw vegetables are encouraged so if you find yourself hungry between meals, eating pre-cut celery, carrots, peppers, cauliflower and broccoli can keep you until you are ready for a meal. Again, integrate the guidelines on nutrition that appears in Chapter 11. Eating healthy foods is a fundamental part of Plan B.

Control Your Portions

Another important element of Plan B is portion control. If you are not counting calories, it is easy to consume too much food, even if the food is healthy. You can easily fool yourself by eating a larger quantity of healthy foods. You might think that you are losing weight, but if you consume too many calories, you can actually gain weight. The problem of quantity has already been touched on, but aside from limiting portions—such as only eating a handful of nuts or one cheese stick—there are other excellent tools that can help. You can control portions by thinking of the food plate again. The food plate provides a way to assure variety, but it can also help in figuring out what a portion size should look like. Take a typical dinner plate. Fill half with fruits and veggies. You need not worry about eating too many fruits and vegetables as they typically have no fat, are generally low in calories, are high in fiber and are healthy. So feel free to load up that side of the plate. Then, fill the other side of the dinner plate with equal portions of protein and carbohydrate.

In Chapter 9 you were guided to estimate calories with your

hands. Now, you are going to measure suitable portions using a similar method. Obviously, it is possible to load a dinner plate to the max, but you are not going to do that. You are to eat reasonable portions. A portion is often equal to a handful. You might take a portion of mashed potatoes that is equivalent to the size of your fist, or grab a dinner roll for your starch instead. A portion of meat should be about the size of your palm, which translates to about 3 ounces. This type of estimation is a learned process. You may find that you are piling the mashed potatoes too high on your plate or not giving yourself enough meat, but most likely, you will catch yourself before you do this because you now know how to estimate portions. You may also use guidelines found on the cans or boxes of prepared foods. If a can of soup says that it contains two portions, eat half. No matter what you put on your plate, eat slowly and tune in to how your body feels. After a while, you will learn how to eat proper portions largely by examining your hunger and fullness levels.

Eat Regular Meals

Come to a routine manner of eating. Rather than eating haphazardly throughout the day, decide on four to six meal times. How do you do this? First, examine how you eat now. Are you eating regular meals? If not, you may be eating healthfully throughout the day, but grazing has the drawback of deceiving your hunger meter. Simply, when you eat small amounts of foods almost constantly throughout the day, you will not feel satisfied. Get into the habit of eating meals. That is, eat vegetables or fruit, some protein, and a small amount of grains at each sitting. You may want to eat just breakfast, lunch, and dinner, but consuming smaller meals throughout the day aids your metabolism. Some of you may not be grazing at all, but find that you eat three rather large meals each day. In fact, some people have a difficult time stopping before they are very full. This behavior is often equated with eating family meals, going to lunch with co-workers, and consuming a lot of food because you know that you will not have the opportunity to eat later in the day. When consuming a lot of food at once, you will not be hungry for a long time, but it is not the most efficient way to eat. You may end up consuming too many calories when you overeat.

The first thing you need to do to fully invest in Plan B is to decide on an eating schedule. Perhaps you want to eat breakfast, lunch, an afternoon snack, dinner, and an evening snack. This is a reasonable goal. Make the decision about when to eat your three to six meals based on your schedule and when you prefer to eat. Keep in mind that a snack is just a meal. However, you may find that in between balanced meals, you want a smaller amount of food. You can refer to these as snacks. Just keep them healthy. Try, as much as possible, to spread your meals evenly throughout the day. Doing so will keep you satiated and is best for your metabolism. Another part of Plan B is to become aware of your hunger and satiety levels. When you are in touch with your hunger, you will naturally fall into a rhythm of eating and abstaining from food.

Are You Plan-B Ready?

If you have read through this chapter, and it sounds good to you, you are Plan-B ready. Simply, eat when you are hungry, and stop eating before you are full. If you eat to fullness, you have already eaten too much. However, if you stop before you are full, your body will be able to use the food properly. Also, eat a variety of healthy foods and eat them at designated meal times. Understanding and incorporating the suggestions in Plan B will see you through a manner of eating where you lose weight without counting calories.

Summary

- ❖ Eat when you are hungry and stop before you are full.
- ❖ Have the goal of eating nutritionally, or as close to nature as possible. Read Chapter 11 for more guidance. Make sure you are committed to healthy eating before you start Plan B.
- ❖ Exercise portion control. Use the plate method to create suitable meals.
- ❖ Eat a variety of foods.
- ❖ Feel free to have unlimited quantities of low calorie vegetables whenever hunger strikes.
- ❖ Eat between four and six meals each day. If you like, some of these may be smaller meals called snacks.
- ❖ This plan is part of a larger program of nutrition, exercise and meditation. In addition to eating in a certain manner, you will be engaging in meditation and exercise.

Notes

CHAPTER 11

EXERCISE, NUTRITION AND MEDITATION

Following an eating plan—either Plan A or Plan B—will help you to create a structure that is comfortable for you, but in order to truly integrate a regimen that will take you successfully through the program and beyond, it is important to understand its three basic components. This program consists of exercise, nutrition, and meditation. If you are knowledgeable about any or all of these elements, you are ahead of the game. If you know very little about them, this chapter will provide you with the necessary information for you to get started on a healthier and stress-free manner of living.

Exercise: Purposeful Movement

In this technologically-oriented time in history, moving your body in a sport or even just in a purposeful fashion is considered exercise. In some other cultures, and certainly before our modern way of life would emerge, people exercised by doing their chores, going to work, and just living their lives. You may say that you do those things too, but you do not have to go out and hunt to put dinner on the table, nor do you have to walk miles to bring water back to your homes. We take modern conveniences—packaged food, plumbing, restaurants—for granted, and while they do bring pleasure to our lives and they leave us time for other pursuits, they create a world where human beings and their animal companions are less likely to move their bodies. When you have to hunt for your dinner, or even if you just have to cook a meal from scratch, there is preparatory time, and energy is utilized. When you eat a couple of slices of pizza quickly so you can get back to the office and sit for another three hours until quitting time, you are hardly expending energy, so you are not burning a lot of calories.

The human body is designed to move, but because as a society we move much less often than our capabilities, we need an outlet to make use of that energy in order to maintain a proper weight and create good health. As a result, gyms have sprung up in many cities. Still, a good number of people do not exercise purposefully at all. Some do, but they may only engage in strenuous physical activity once a week or less. Of course, everyone has 168 hours per week at their disposal, so there is ample time to engage in purposeful, targeted exercises. If we exercise just one hour per day, that hour is only a small percentage of our total available hours. In fact, if we were to exercise each day for just sixty minutes, we would still have 161 hours left in our weeks to do other things. Plus, devoting one hour per day each week to exercise will make a tremendous difference in our lives. Yet, many people would find spending sixty minutes each day engaged in purposeful movement rather difficult. Why? They get into routines where they are not moving very much, so suddenly devoting a block of time each day to activity can be challenging and this is understandable. If you have not been moving much, getting in that hour seems exhausting and it would be if you dove in headfirst. How do you get through your first few days or weeks of exercise? Adding exercise gradually is the answer.

The instruction contained in this book includes a program that allows you to gradually add exercise to your day. Three days per week, you will do 15 minutes of stretching along with cardiovascular exercise that is often referred to simply as cardio. Cardio—exercise that works your heart and lungs—can be whatever cardiovascular exercise you choose. Consider different types of activities. Examples of cardio or aerobic activity are walking, hiking, jogging, golfing, kayaking, downhill skiing, swimming, jumping rope, cycling, rock climbing and high impact aerobics. If you join a gym, you will be able to meet your aerobics quota on the treadmill, the stationary bicycle or the elliptical machine. Even if you do join a gym, you might want to mix and match activities. For example, you may want to make use of the elliptical machine at the gym one day, but ride the bicycle path outdoors another day. Also, many fitness centers include a variety of aerobic classes like Zumba, spin, and various types of boot camps. The more you vary the type of aerobic exercise, the stronger your body will be, and the more calories you will burn. This is good because your body gets used to certain activities and burns calories at a certain level, but when you change the activity, you surprise your body, and it shifts into high gear. However, you need not do something different all the time. Perhaps you run outdoors or on the treadmill for three weeks. Then, after that, you take a water aerobics class for a few weeks, and then, you buy a mountain bike and try that out. The point is, vary your activity over time and you will be rewarded with a metabolism that doesn't quit.

The first week of the cardio program is only equivalent to 15 minutes, so that first week you will stretch for 15 minutes and then do whatever cardio exercise you enjoy for only 15 minutes. You may want to take a walk or something similar just to get the feel for moving your body. As the weeks go on, the cardio gradually increases until you are up to 40 minutes on cardio days. At that point, you are engaging in an ideal amount of exercise. On alternate days, you simply do a weight training routine. An example of a typical routine is provided in the pages that follow.

This program is based on generally accepted standards of exercise and is in line with recommendations of the American College of Sports Medicine (ACSM). Once you are in the maintenance phase of the program, you will be physically fit, but if you want to add more exercise, that is fine too. Add activities you enjoy. You might want to train for a half marathon, or go rock climbing, or go for a long hike in the mountains. If you already consider yourself fairly active and the program is so easy for you that you want to add more activities, you may wonder about overdoing it. You likely do not need to be concerned, but do exercise caution and consult a medical professional before engaging in extremely strenuous activities.

Exercise probably accelerates weight loss more than anything else, so if you become extraordinarily active, you probably will not have a weight issue. Why? When you exercise, you use calories. But it is not only burning calories that helps you lose weight. When you exercise, you alter your metabolism and so your body functions more efficiently. As time goes on, you will see a noticeable change in not only your weight, but in your shape. If you lose weight without exercise—something difficult to do but possible—you will not reap the enormous benefits that you otherwise would such as gaining muscle, toning your body, and using food more efficiently. When you are exercising, losing and maintaining weight is much easier.

What you probably do not realize now is that once you start exercising, you will gain energy and have a more efficient metabolism. Athletes have a lot of energy and burn a lot of calories. They may spend time training several hours per day, but imagine how much they accomplish because of the energy boost they feel when their body works efficiently! You will also be much more satisfied psychologically and emotionally. Exercise is good for anxiety and depression. It lowers blood pressure. It can help resolve sleep problems. So when you worry about the fact that exercising is time consuming, think of your life in terms of energy expenditure, and not just in terms of linear time. You will sleep better, and you will get much more accomplished when you are physically fit than if you sat at your desk for that hour you think you need.

Interestingly, ACSM claims that even if you follow their guidelines, it does not make up for a sedentary lifestyle. In other words, even if you implement a suitable exercise program and feel as if you are in great shape, it does not mean that sitting most of the day is healthy. In fact, ACSM claims that a sedentary lifestyle is a health risk factor in and of itself. Many people are tied to their desks, so it is not uncommon to see people sit for long periods of time. Does this mean you have to exercise for an hour and actually engage in other physical activity too? Yes, but it's really not hard, and it will come naturally. Right now, you may be lying on the couch thinking that you could not possibly exercise for an hour each day, and then try to move even more, but your thinking will change once you start the plan.

There are many things you can do to add movement to your day. If you have a desk job, take a walk during your lunch hour, take the stairs instead of the elevator, and do chores at home instead of sitting in front of the television the entire evening. You might want to engage in scheduled activities after dinner, a plan that will not only get you to move a little bit more, but will make it less likely that you will want to eat. And if you think this sounds daunting, don't worry. Once you are in shape, you will *want* to move. Again, you will gain more energy and you will be bursting at the seams looking for something active to do, seriously.

In summary, your exercise equation is simply to follow the guidelines in this book. There is little to think about if you follow the simple plan provided, but you will need to make choices when it comes to aerobic activity. You may also want to use a different weight training routine, which is fine. The routine provided is simply an example. The time you invest for each type of exercise is outlined for you in a gradual way so you become accustomed to moving. You may find it difficult to make the change at first, but remember, you can change a habit with perseverance. Exercise will soon become a satisfying part of your life. Our bodies were made to move and when you give your body what it wants, you will be encouraging it to assume a more desirable and healthier state.

The Exercise Plan

The exercise suggestions contained in the pages that follow include workouts to be done over the course of eight weeks time. The workouts are provided in the charts contained in the next several pages, and a description of each exercise is included in the exercise description section that follows the plan. You may choose to follow the program to the letter, or you may want to work with a personal trainer. How you approach exercise is strictly up to you. We offer these suggestions as they are basic movements used by many trainers. In fact, you may want to explore the movements further, and additional variations, by reading books devoted to training, watching videos on YouTube, or working with a fitness professional. Each of the exercises described will tone or strengthen your muscles. The exercise progressions that appear in this book is for the purpose of teaching a novice about exercise, but it in no way represents the enormous variety of resources that can help you get into shape.

There are some things that are important to know before you begin to exercise. When you are doing the workouts, make sure to tighten your core before each exercise. This means you tighten your trunk. A good way to be sure you are doing this correctly is to imagine that someone is going to punch you in the stomach. What do you do? To lighten the impact you automatically tighten your core. It is second nature. A tight core is important for every single exercise you do. Your core supports your vital organs. When you tighten your core, you are able to strengthen the main part of your body so the rest of it does not have to work as hard. The core is your powerhouse. It is the foundation of your physical body. When you properly tighten your core before you begin each of the exercises, you also reduce your chances of injury. Another important thing to keep in mind before beginning each exercise is to breathe properly. Breathe out on the contraction, and breathe in when you are releasing the contraction. You should exhale and inhale once for each repetition. When you exercise, always think about your core and your breathing. This cannot be emphasized enough.

If you choose to follow the recommendations contained in this chapter, engage in the workouts for two weeks before you move on to the next two-week phase. The final workout plan is also considered a maintenance plan. You can continue to use this program indefinitely, but you will want to tweak it a bit over time. Any program you engage in should be changed frequently because your body gets used to a certain training routine and once it does, your body will not change as quickly. The goal is to continually challenge your body.

We suggest that you increase your aerobic activity over time from 15 to 40 minutes, and on the three days each week you focus on aerobics, apply a flexibility regimen. On alternate days, do engage in weight training exercises. In a typical week, you might want to do aerobic and flexibility activities on Monday, Wednesday and Friday, and then on Tuesday, Thursday and Saturday engage in the weight strengthening routine.

Before you begin, you will need to find a place to perform the exercises. You can do these exercises just about anywhere. If you choose to exercise at a fitness center, the facility will likely contain the equipment you need. If you do them at home, you will need to purchase a few inexpensive items such as dumbbells and an elastic workout band. You will also find that an exercise mat on a hard floor provides the most comfort for engaging in the routines.

After you begin, you will notice that this program increases gradually in terms of the level of difficulty. Again, you will be exercising for six days each week, incorporating cardio and flexibility every other day, and on alternate days you will do the strength training routines provided.

Weeks 1 and 2

Flexibility and Cardio: 3 days per week

Flexibility: 15 Minutes. When performing these stretches, hold each pose for about 30 seconds. Feel free to add your own exercises.

Hamstring: Stand up. Bend over and try to touch your toes.

Hip flexor and calf: With one foot forward bend your knee at a 90-degree angle and allow the other leg to straighten behind you. Repeat on the other side.

Side to side: Stand straight. Bend over on one side of your body and grab your ankle with one hand. Rest the other hand on the wrist of the hand holding your ankle. Repeat on the other side.

Chest and shoulders: From a standing position, clasp your hands behind you, reach out, and stretch.

Upper back: From a standing position, clasp your hands in front of you. Then, round your back while pushing forward and stretch.

Neck: Keeping your body straight, move your head to the left and then to the right. Then slowly move your ear to one shoulder, and then to the other. Do both of these movements slowly. Repeat 5 times on each side.

Cardio: 15 minutes, 3 days per week along with flexibility. Choose from a variety of exercises such as walking, jogging, cycling, jumping rope, swimming, rowing, or taking an aerobics class.

Training: 3 days per week

Pilates Bridge	4 poses	20 seconds each pose
Long Arm Crunch	2 sets	12 repetitions
Waist Oblique I	2 sets	12 repetitions
Core Balance/ Bird Dog	2 sets	12 repetitions
Incline Push Ups	2 sets	12 repetitions
Wall Squat	2 sets	12 repetitions
Standing Row with resistance band	2 sets	12 repetitions

Weeks 3 and 4

Flexibility and Cardio: 3 days per week

Flexibility: 15 Minutes. When performing these stretches, hold each pose for about 30 seconds. Feel free to add your own exercises.

Hamstring: Stand up. Bend over and try to touch your toes.

Hip flexor and calf: With one foot forward bend your knee at a 90-degree angle and allow the other leg to straighten behind you. Repeat on the other side.

Side to side: Stand straight. Bend over on one side of your body and grab your ankle with one hand. Rest the other hand on the wrist of the hand holding your ankle. Repeat on the other side.

Chest and shoulders: From a standing position, clasp your hands behind you, reach out, and stretch.

Upper back: From a standing position, clasp your hands in front of you. Then, round your back while pushing forward and stretch.

Neck: Keeping your body straight, move your head to the left and then to the right. Then slowly move your ear to one shoulder, and then to the other. Do both of these movements slowly. Repeat 5 times on each side.

Cardio: 20 minutes, 3 days per week along with flexibility. Choose from a variety of exercises such as walking, jogging, cycling, jumping rope, swimming, rowing, or taking an aerobics class.

Training: 3 days per week

Pilates Bridge	4 poses	20 seconds each pose
Long Arm Crunch	3 sets	15 repetitions
Waist Oblique I	3 sets	15 repetitions
Core Balance/ Bird Dog	3 sets	15 repetitions
Incline Push Ups	3 sets	12 repetitions
Chair Squat	3 sets	15 repetitions
Standing Row with resistance band	3 sets	15 repetitions

Weeks 5 and 6

Flexibility and Cardio: 3 days per week

Flexibility: 15 Minutes. When performing these stretches, hold each pose for about 30 seconds. Feel free to add your own exercises.

Hamstring: Stand up. Bend over and try to touch your toes.

Hip flexor and calf: With one foot forward bend your knee at a 90-degree angle and allow the other leg to straighten behind you. Repeat on the other side.

Side to side: Stand straight. Bend over on one side of your body and grab your ankle with one hand. Rest the other hand on the wrist of the hand holding your ankle. Repeat on the other side.

Chest and shoulders: From a standing position, clasp your hands behind you, reach out, and stretch.

Upper back: From a standing position, clasp your hands in front of you. Then, round your back while pushing forward and stretch.

Neck: Keeping your body straight, move your head to the left and then to the right. Then slowly move your ear to one shoulder, and then to the other. Do both of these movements slowly. Repeat 5 times on each side.

Cardio: 25 minutes, 3 days per week along with flexibility. Choose from a variety of exercises such as walking, jogging, cycling, jumping rope, swimming, rowing, or taking an aerobics class.

Training: 3 days per week

Plank	4 poses	20 seconds each pose
Superman I	2 sets	8 repetitions
Waist Oblique II	2 sets	12 repetitions
Bicycle Crunch	2 sets	12 repetitions
Push Ups on Knees	2 sets	12 repetitions
Squat (with or without free weights)	2 sets	12 repetitions
Bent Over Row (with free weights)	2 sets	8 repetitions

Weeks 7 and 8

Flexibility and Cardio: 3 days per week

Flexibility: 15 Minutes. When performing these stretches, hold each pose for about 30 seconds. Feel free to add your own exercises.

Hamstring: Stand up. Bend over and try to touch your toes.

Hip flexor and calf: With one foot forward bend your knee at a 90-degree angle and allow the other leg to straighten behind you. Repeat on the other side.

Side to side: Stand straight. Bend over on one side of your body and grab your ankle with one hand. Rest the other hand on the wrist of the hand holding your ankle. Repeat on the other side.

Chest and shoulders: From a standing position, clasp your hands behind you, reach out, and stretch.

Upper back: From a standing position, clasp your hands in front of you. Then, round your back while pushing forward and stretch.

Neck: Keeping your body straight, move your head to the left and then to the right. Then slowly move your ear to one shoulder, and then to the other. Do both of these movements slowly. Repeat 5 times on each side.

Cardio: 30 minutes, 3 days per week along with flexibility. Choose from a variety of exercises such as walking, jogging, cycling, jumping rope, swimming, rowing, or taking an aerobics class.

Training: 3 days per week

Plank	5 poses	30 seconds each pose
Superman I	2 sets	8 repetitions
Superman II	5 poses	20 seconds each pose
Single Leg Balance Reach	2 sets	12 repetitions
Bicycle Crunch	3 sets	15 repetitions
Push Ups on Knees	3 sets	15 repetitions
Split Squat Lunges (with or without free weights)	3 sets	15 repetitions
Bent Over Row (with free weights)	3 sets	12 repetitions

Maintenance Phase
Flexibility and Cardio: 3 days per week

Flexibility: 15 Minutes. When performing these stretches, hold each pose for about 30 seconds. Feel free to add your own exercises.

Hamstring: Stand up. Bend over and try to touch your toes.

Hip flexor and calf: With one foot forward bend your knee at a 90-degree angle and allow the other leg to straighten behind you. Repeat on the other side.

Side to side: Stand straight. Bend over on one side of your body and grab your ankle with one hand. Rest the other hand on the wrist of the hand holding your ankle. Repeat on the other side.

Chest and shoulders: From a standing position, clasp your hands behind you, reach out, and stretch.

Upper back: From a standing position, clasp your hands in front of you. Then, round your back while pushing forward and stretch.

Neck: Keeping your body straight, move your head to the left and then to the right. Then slowly move your ear to one shoulder, and then to the other. Do both of these movements slowly. Repeat 5 times on each side.

Cardio: 40 minutes, 3 days per week along with flexibility. Choose from a variety of exercises such as walking, jogging, cycling, jumping rope, swimming, rowing, or taking an aerobics class.

Training: 3 days per week

Plank	5 poses	30 seconds each pose
Plank (Mountain Climber Variation)	3 sets	1 minute
Plank (Leg Abduction Variation)	1 set	1 minute (30 seconds on each side)
Push Ups	2 sets	10 repetitions
Abs	3 sets	15 repetitions
Reverse Crunches	3 sets	15 repetitions
Lunges	3 sets	15 repetitions
Side Squat	3 sets	15 repetitions
Military Press (with free weights)	3 sets	15 repetitions

Exercise Descriptions

Abs: Lie on your back with your legs up and your arms on the ground above your head. Touch your toes with your hands. Repeat the movement for the desired amount of repetitions.

Bent Over Row: With one dumbbell in hand, put your opposite knee and hand on the seat of a chair. Bend your elbow, bringing the dumbbell up to your chest and then bring it back down. Repeat the movement for the desired amount of repetitions. Perform this exercise slowly. **Note**: Start with 8 lb. dumbbells (free weights). If they are too heavy, lower the weight as much as you need. Increase to 10 lb. weights when you are ready.

Core Balance/ Bird Dog: Get on your hands and knees and reach one arm in front of you while you extend the opposite back leg. Balance your body with the arm and leg that is still on the ground. Then switch sides. Keep repeating for the specified number of reps.

Crunches: Lie down on your back with your knees bent. With hands supporting your head, lift shoulders off the floor, while assuring that your core is tight and that your lower back remains firm against the floor. Repeat the movement for the desired amount of repetitions. For the *Long Arm Crunch,* lie down on your back with your knees bent. With arms over your head, lift shoulders off the floor, while assuring that your core is tight and that your lower back remains firm against the floor. Repeat the movement for the desired amount of repetitions. For the *Bicycle Crunch*, start with your arms behind your head. You engage in movement by alternating your legs as if you are riding a bicycle, bringing your opposite elbow to your knees for each repetition. For a *Reverse Crunch*, lie down with your arms alongside your body, bringing your legs up as straight as possible. While keeping your back on the floor, point your toes and attempt to touch the ceiling with your feet. Repeat the movement for the desired amount of repetitions.

Lunge: Placing one foot forward, move your body in a downward motion, bending your front knee and lifting the heel of your back leg slightly off the floor. Be sure that your torso is straight, that your back knee is also bent, and that your front leg does not go past your toes. Repeat for the desired number of repetitions.

Military Press: Stand with your legs shoulder width apart. Pick up two dumbbells and start at the shoulder level. Stretch your arms straight above your head, and then bring the weights back down, bending your elbows so that the weights come back to your shoulders. Complete the movement for the desired amount of repetitions. **Note:** Start with 8 lb. dumbbells (free weights). If they are too heavy, lower the weight. Increase to 10 lb. weights when you are ready.

Pilates Bridge: Lie on the floor, on your back, with your knees bent, while your feet rest on the floor. Squeeze your glutes, while slowly lifting your pelvis, keeping your shoulders on the floor. The pose essentially creates a triangle with your body. Hold the pose. Repeat and hold the position for the desired amount of poses.

Plank: For the regular plank, lie down on the floor on your stomach. Place your forearms on the floor, and squeeze your glutes. Then lift your body so your arms are perpendicular to the floor but your forearm remains snug to the ground. With this pose, your entire body forms a straight line. *The Mountain Climber* variation begins in the plank position, supporting yourself on your hands. However, the left knee is bent, and the left foot is lifted from the floor. The pose is repeated with the right leg. Continue to switch legs rapidly so it appears as if you are climbing stairs. The *Leg Abduction* variation is when you are in the plank position, but where one leg moves away from your body. Move the leg out, and bring it back in for the desired number of repetitions.

Push Ups: The traditional push up sees you facing the ground. Before you begin, tighten your core and glutes. As you stretch your arms, your body is elevated and in line with the ground. Move your body up and down, keeping your back straight, while bending your elbows. A variation of the push up is to perform the exercise on your knees. For *Push Ups on knees,* do the same thing, but instead of lifting your entire body up, rest on your knees and only lift your body from the hips up. Finally, an *Incline Push Up* is a push up, except your hands rest on a kitchen counter or another high surface, or even a wall.

Single Leg Balance Reach: Stand with arms along your body. Then, lean forward with one arm stretched in front of you, reaching for the ground, and the opposite leg lifted behind you. Squeeze your glutes and return to the standing position.

Standing Row with resistance band: Use your resistance band. Wrap it around a sturdy pole, but make sure that you are standing an arm's distance away. Your arms and elbows should be straight. Begin by pulling the band so your elbows are slowly brought back to your sides. Reach your arms straight out in front of you, and pull back again. Each pull back is a rep. Repeat the movement for the desired amount of repetitions.

Squats: A *Wall Squat* is done starting in a standing position. Lean against the wall with your back pressed flat against it. Bend your knees and squat down as you follow the wall. A *Chair Squat* sees you begin in a sitting position where you raise yourself out of the chair. *Split Squat Lunges* sees you begin standing, and then lunging with each leg alternately. To perform this exercise with dumbbells, do split squat lunges while holding one dumbbell in each hand. For *Side Squats*, begin standing and move your leg to the left. Then squat. Repeat on the right. Continue to alternate left and right positions.

Superman : Superman exercises are done lying on the ground. For *Superman I*, begin in this position, with your stomach on the floor. Alternate arms and legs by moving your left arm and right leg up, while keeping alternate arms and legs down on the ground. Repeat on the other side. For *Superman II*, simply reach your arms and legs up in front and behind you off the ground so you look like Superman did when he was flying. Hold this pose.

Waist Obliques: For the *Waist Oblique I*, lie down on the floor on your back, with your knees up to your chest. Roll the lower part of your body from side to side. For the *Waist Oblique II*, lie down on the floor with your knees up against your chest and roll from side to side in such a way that your knees and arms are always on the opposite sides of your body.

By the time you arrive at week 9, you will begin the maintenance phase. You will continue to do at least 40 minutes of aerobics and flexibility training three times per week, as well as weight resistance training on alternate days. Plan to rest on the seventh day. Combined with 10 minutes of meditation, you will be taking just about an hour each day for yourself on most days. And remember, you are worth it!

Nutrition

Nutrition on some level is common sense. We all know that certain foods are good for us, and we know what should be labeled "junk food." We know that carrots and cauliflower are low in calories and full of nutrients but that snack cakes and doughnuts are riddled with saturated fat and sugar. But what is really important to know is that there are no bad foods, not really. There are of course objectively unhealthy foods. When you are educated about food, and know what it does to your body, you will have the tools to make intelligent choices so if you choose to eat a snack cake, you will do so consciously, without guilt, and rarely. Once you are educated, you will probably not be eating unhealthy foods daily. However, making peace with food is important to the process. It means that others are free to eat whatever they want around you, and you will not be rattled when you see something unhealthy in your environment. Nothing is forbidden. At the same time, nothing you really want is in the cookie jar.

That said, in a broad diet that includes variety, there is room for a doughnut on occasion, and in fact, there is nothing wrong with eating some things that diet gurus have told us are unhealthy. The bagel for example gets a bad rap because it contains a lot of calories in proportion to other seeming equivalents like a slice of white toast. Caloric intake is important when you are trying to lose weight, but another reason why the bagel is considered junk food is due to the "empty" calories it contains and the fact that it is made largely of carbohydrate. Eating an overabundance of simple carbohydrates, even if consumed in a desirable caloric range, is inconsistent with a healthy, balanced diet.

Before going on to dismantle the bagel, and rebuild it to nutritional desirability, a look at calories is in order. Plan A prompts you to count calories. Everything you have known about dieting in the past is tied to calorie counting. So what is a calorie anyway? First, when we refer to calories in everyday vernacular we are technically referring to kilocalories, which is a unit of heat. As units of heat or energy, calories are needed to provide the energy to drive the human body in all of its functions. Even if you just sat around all day, you need a certain amount of calories at a minimum for your body to function in a healthy manner, and not all calories are created equal. Proteins and carbohydrate contain about 4 calories for each gram consumed, while fat is equivalent to about 9 calories per gram. That is why there are 100 calories in a tablespoon of butter even though it seems to be a very small portion of food. Now, back to the bagel. A bagel is made largely of carbohydrate, but it is a bit larger, and denser, than a slice of bread. It has too many carbohydrates for it to be considered good for you, so how can you eat the bagel and consider yourself eating well?

First, a bagel is just a bagel. It is not inherently bad or bad for you. But consider this: bagels and toast come in different varieties. If you can get your hands on a whole grain bagel, for example, it is high in fiber, something that turns the bad old bagel into a decent breakfast. For example, the Dunkin Donuts Multigrain Bagel contains about 330 calories. If you eat just half, smeared with a reduced fat Laughing Cow cheese spread, you have approximately 200 calories that you may count towards your breakfast calorie ration. From that part of the meal, you also get about 5 grams of fiber, and if you add a piece of fruit or a yogurt, you have a breakfast that will help your weight loss effort. If you missed it, the key point is that you are eating only half of the bagel so you reduce the calories and carbs substantially.

The bagel with cheese and fruit is a satisfying breakfast but even if you love it, don't eat it every day. When you eat the same things daily, not only will you get bored, but you will also miss out on nutrients you could glean by eating a variety of foods. You could have a half a bagel and fruit one day, then the next day eat a bowl of oatmeal with a sprinkle of fresh blueberries, a cup of coffee, and a soft boiled egg. Vary your meals, and you will begin to understand what it is like to enjoy fresh foods again, and don't be afraid to get adventurous. Go to the fruit and vegetable section in your local grocery store and buy something you never heard of, or find new, healthy recipes and cook something fabulous. Decide to change up your food choices, and remember the French way of eating, which is to enjoy healthy foods in a leisurely fashion.

Eating food that is closest to nature, the La Leche League nutritional philosophy, is a good foundation when designing a healthy food plan. In fact, many nutritionists say that people should shop around the perimeter of the store, leaving the aisles of prepared food alone. Indeed, the best foods for you are the fresh varieties. Of course, in today's harried society, many people do not take the time to cook, so there are aisles and aisles of packaged foods available. You may be consuming more of these foods than you like because you feel you are already short on time and resist cooking meals from scratch. If you do feel too stressed for time to cook, your lifestyle may be one of the areas you want to re-examine. Remember, you are changing your thinking, and changing the parts of your life that are not working. You will be devoting an hour a day to taking care of yourself with exercise and meditation. Also, devote an hour a week to rethinking your food choices. Plan menus and create your shopping list. Once you have the ingredients in the house, cooking may become one of your greatest pleasures. And think about this: when you are cooking, you are standing, moving, stirring, flipping and all the while burning calories. You are participating in your meals rather than using an electric appliance to quickly heat food that probably has way too much salt and lacks the nutrition that only fresh foods contain.

Certainly, you can find a few minutes to sauté chicken breasts while boiling water to blanch your green beans, where you will have a healthy meal rather quickly. And when you do take more time to cook something grand, double the recipe and freeze some for another day. Eating raw or cold foods can also be satisfying and nutritious and these dishes do not take very long to prepare. A quick fix is to throw everything into a salad from leftover chicken to hard cooked eggs, spritz it with an oil and vinegar dressing, and voila, you have a healthy lunch or dinner. Simply choose the freshest and healthiest ingredients you prefer and be creative in coming up with simple meal strategies. Do plan ahead by deciding what you will cook when so that you will be prepared. But if you are really in a rush, driving through a fast food window need not derail your plan. Order a salad with a low calorie dressing, or select another option such as a grilled chicken sandwich. There are ways to eat healthier no matter where you are. Just make it a point to move toward fresher and healthier foods.

The basics of nutrition are somewhat simple, but there are details that you need to know. When it comes to healthy eating, the concept of fat content is an important one to grasp. Read the labels and check nutrition counters. Ideally, never eat anything containing trans fat. That type of fat is considered to be so bad for you that cities like New York have actually banned it from their restaurants. Monounsaturated and polyunsaturated fats, on the other hand, are healthy. Saturated fat however is not so good. It is implicated in raising blood cholesterol levels so ideally, minimize this kind of fat. While total fat count is good to know, you will primarily be looking to see how much saturated fat is in an item per serving. But keep in mind, when an item does have a high fat content—even if it is low in saturated fat—it is likely to be high in calories.

What is a high saturated fat count? When looking at fat grams, numbers will range from zero to double digits. It is best to keep the number low. The American Heart Association recommends that people not eat more than 7% of their total calories in saturated fats. It is possible to calculate how many saturated fat grams you would ideally eat based on how many calories you consume, but counting both saturated fat grams and calories would be tedious. An easier way to look at saturated fat is to evaluate each food that comes your way. Rather than eating an abundance of fat-free foods along with some that contain a lot of fat, it makes sense to evaluate each item for fat content. A good rule of thumb is not to eat products containing more than 3 or 4 grams of saturated fat per serving. This is not difficult because there are many tasty food choices that have less than 4 grams of fat. Even a regular fast food hamburger makes the cut at 3.5 grams.

When you make choices, you will weigh more factors than the amount of fat grams. The example of the fast food hamburger helps to illustrate that point. That is, if the hamburger fits the fat content requirement, why not eat it? You can, and you probably will on occasion, but the truth is that the regular hamburger is very small and for 250 calories, you could have had something much more substantial. The burger contains fat so it is relatively high in calories for its size. The bun is made of carbohydrate, but not the good kind. So there is little to fill you up. And if you have fries with that, you would be eating the equivalent of almost two meals in respect to calorie count, not to mention an excessive amount of fat. You can eat the small hamburger that is, by the way, the main ingredient of a child's meal, but then you might be hungry. So if you find yourself in a fast food restaurant, the salad is a much better calorie and nutrition choice. In McDonald's, for example, a premium Caesar salad with grilled chicken is only 190 calories. Newman's Own low fat balsamic vinaigrette is only 35 calories. For slightly less calories than the restaurant's smallest burger, you can eat a delicious salad that will keep you satisfied until your next meal.

When you begin to think about nutrition, you will realize that certain foods will not make you fat necessarily, but they won't serve you well. You want to eat nutritiously, feel satisfied, and gain energy from the food you eat. Therefore, there are a number of other things you will want to consider. You already know how to evaluate fat content. You want the healthy fats, and you want to avoid the unhealthy ones, but there is another very important factor in eating healthy, and that is to examine sugar content. It is also important to know what type of sugar is in your food. Some processed foods are somewhat high in sugar but they may still be nutritious if they are sweetened with fruit. The sugars that are in fruit still have a deleterious effect on your body as does granulated sugar and high fructose corn syrup, but gravitating toward fruit juice sweeteners and honey and pure maple syrup will certainly take you on a more natural path to eating. Also, when you are eating an apple or orange for example, you are absorbing vitamins and getting fiber from the snack. When you are eating something with added sugar, you are eating something that contains unnecessary sweeteners. The extra sugar adds calories and it takes a toll on the body. Although natural sugars are more desirable than the artificial kind, all sugars have the same effect on the body. Sugar is a carbohydrate. Blood glucose rises in response to eating carbs, and this causes insulin to be released. While this is a normal bodily response, an overabundance of carbohydrates will prompt your body to work overtime.

When looking at grams of sugar contained in a product, do consider whether the sugar is derived from fruit sources and also consider the overall health of the product. Then compare the labels. There are cereals that contain only 3 grams of sugar and others that have 23, so when selecting a product, look for items with the least amount of sugar. Ideally, select products with 5 grams of sugar per serving or less. Also, gravitate towards sugar that comes from natural sources. Keep in mind that some healthy products such as Kashi's Blackberry Graham Soft-Baked Cereal Bar have more than 5 grams of sugar. While higher than the recommended 5 grams perhaps, the healthy ingredients make up for the additional 2 grams of sugar. The bar has 3 grams of fiber, and fiber is something that is highly desirable for proper digestive functioning. Plus, it contains zero grams of saturated fat. When looking at the ingredients, the Kashi bar seems healthier than other types of cereal bars on the market. This particular bar is sweetened with pear and cane juices and molasses for example, as opposed to high fructose corn syrup that is a sweetener in some competitive brands.

Artificial sweeteners have been viewed as something that

on some level resolves the problem of eating too much sugar, but conflicting studies put its safety in doubt. Using sugar from natural sources in moderation, and artificial sweeteners on occasion, will help you to move toward a balanced, healthy diet. Getting used to foods that are less sweet takes time, but reducing sugar is often recommended by doctors and nutritionists. Of course, few foods are perfectly nutritious, containing the recommended amount of saturated fat, fiber, and sugar. But do read the labels. Your food choices should, on balance, be healthy. If you are counting calories, you do not have to concern yourself with nutrition if your only goal is to lose weight. You are counting calories for the day and you can eat whatever you like. However, because you want to do what is best for your body, you will want to choose healthy options, and when you do, you will experience a reduced amount of hunger. If you are not counting calories, you do have to be careful about consuming calorie dense foods that may not fill you up quickly. Nuts are high in calories, and while they are high in fat, they contain healthy fats. Yet, too many nuts or too many peanut butter sandwiches can add calories very quickly, so being aware of high calorie content will help you to decide portion size. Further, even if you do eat a lot of cashews one evening, don't fret. If you are eating a variety of healthy foods, it will hardly matter. When you choose variety, things will naturally even out.

So far, you learned what to avoid, but there are things you will want to include. It is important to incorporate sufficient protein in the diet. Consume at least 5 ounces of protein. You also want to assure that you are getting adequate vitamins, and drinking enough water. A daily multi-vitamin may not be enough to create optimal health. You may want to consult a health care professional who can make recommendations geared to your body specifically. Water is very important too. It aids digestion, and actually can accelerate weight loss. As you exercise more, your body will let you know when it is time to drink. Once you are thirsty, you are already dehydrated, so it is prudent to drink water prophylactically. The old adage of drinking eight glasses of water is probably good advice, but you may find you require more than that when you start working out. It is hard to drink too much water unless you are participating in a water drinking game—something that is very dangerous—or you have kidney problems. Otherwise, your level of thirst and the color of your urine-it should be light yellow-can be your guide to determine if you are well hydrated. Finally, adequate fiber aids digestion and may help to prevent cancer. Fiber is simply a type of carbohydrate that the body is incapable of digesting. Most women should aim for at least 20 grams of fiber each day. You can easily obtain enough fiber in your diet by eating fruit, vegetables, cereal, nuts and legumes. While fiber is a carbohydrate, unlike some other types, it actually helps to prevent insulin resistance.

Do include variety in your food selections. Your food choices should be relatively low in saturated fat and sugar, but they should also be tasty and desirable. You do not want to get into the habit of choosing foods that only meet the guidelines set here to the letter, nor do you want to eat some "good" foods and only eat "bad" foods on occasion. The foods themselves are not inherently aligned with morality. Some good foods will not necessarily fit the saturated fat or sugar criteria suggested, but they have a place in a well-rounded diet. The key is to choose wholesome, nutritious foods you enjoy most of the time, as well as other foods that are easily available to you. This means that if you end up going to a restaurant without time to prepare, order a lean cut of meat and ask if they will substitute a vegetable for the potato, or order a salad with the dressing on the side. There is nothing wrong with the potato—it is a vegetable—but it is a carbohydrate and when adding butter and sour cream, the calorie and fat count escalates. Similarly, dressing is fine on a salad, but too much translates to a lot of calories. Whether or not you are counting calories, this type of conscious and conscientious evaluation will help you feel satiated and is a healthy way of living.

Integrating nutrition into your daily diet is a process. You will not learn how to eat healthy overnight. There are numerous ways of learning about nutrition including reading books, watching educational television programs, taking a course at a local community college, or making an appointment with a nutritionist. Your interest in nutrition will help you to make daily food choices, but the basics have already been provided for you. Make the focal point of your diet fruit, vegetables, lean meats, low fat dairy products, and whole grains. They are the ingredients of a healthy diet. Make sure to include healthy monounsaturated and polyunsaturated fats that are found in nuts and seeds. Herbs and spices should make all of your choices palatable. Shop the perimeter of the supermarket for the ingredients. Pay attention to labels and particularly to the grams of sugar and saturated fat, as well as the specific listed ingredients. The fewer the ingredients, the more natural the product probably is. Again, healthier sweeteners are found closer to nature such as pure maple syrup, honey, and stevia. In general, the more you can reduce the use of sugar and artificial sweeteners, the better it is for you, but as with anything else, wean yourself gradually. The research on fat is clearer. Healthy fats are the monounsaturated fats and polyunsaturated fats. Cut out trans fats. Minimize saturated fats. Include enough protein, fiber and water, and do make sure you are getting a sufficient amount of vitamins. Eat a variety of foods, and use the food plate method you learned about in Chapter 10. Those are the basic, generally accepted guidelines. Of course, there is no one rule for determining what is a healthy food and what is not. Use your knowledge, your intuition, and your common sense to eat well every day.

Nutrition Summary

❖ Take one hour each week to plan your menus and shopping lists.

❖ Shop the perimeter of the food store and eat foods that are as close to nature as possible.

❖ Trans fats should be eliminated. Saturated fats should be no more than 4 grams per serving most of the time.

❖ When sweetening your food, or eating sweets, note the source of the sugar. Is it from a natural source? Either way, most of the time, eat items that have no more than 5 grams of sugar per serving. Choose products with artificial sweeteners rarely.

❖ Try to include at least 5 ounces of protein in your daily diet.

❖ Try to include at least 20 grams of fiber in your daily diet.

❖ Do take vitamins, drink enough water, and eat a variety of foods.

❖ Foods are not inherently good or bad, but some foods are much healthier than other foods.

❖ No food is forbidden, but it is wise to focus attention on healthy foods and eat unhealthy food rarely.

❖ Enjoy cooking, eat small amounts of a variety of healthy foods, and savor every bite.

Meditation

Meditation is something that is discussed a lot today. Even in this stress-laden culture where few people stop to rest, doctors have praised alternative modalities such as biofeedback and yoga, suggesting that breathing is a way to relax and lower blood pressure. Meditation is not just one thing. There are different forms of meditation. Some types of meditation require complete quiet and stillness, while others include rhythmic movements. Walking through a labyrinth or meditation garden can be relaxing as can four-square breathing, a method of breath work recommended by medical professionals to reduce anxiety. All of the named modalities include attention to the breath, which is the basis of most types of meditation.

While there are many forms, the basics include being quiet, breathing, and being present. Meditation takes you into the now, so while thoughts about the past and the future come into your consciousness, you can let them go. You need not try to clear your mind completely. That is impossible. Notice your thoughts, but do not feed them. In other words, just notice that you are thinking and let the thoughts leave as quickly as they came in. One technique that guards against intrusive thoughts is to count your breaths. Other ways to meditate include focusing your attention on a part of your body or on an object, such as a flickering candle. When you place your awareness on something that exists in the present, you become more focused on the now, and less on the past and the future.

If you are relaxed, breathing and sitting quietly with your eyes closed, you begin to feel that you are all there is. Everything else is outside of your body and you may experience the feeling that nothing else matters. You will begin to forget about the overdue library book, the speech you have to give at work tomorrow, and the pimple that just will not go away. When you are still, you connect with the inner part of yourself. Learning that this is possible will eventually transform your life. Meditation need not take a lot of time, and while you are not required to do a full lotus to reap the benefits of the altered state of consciousness, keeping your spine straight allows you to inhale deeply and will prevent you from falling asleep.

Just as there are numerous nutrition and exercise books and DVDs on the market, there are wonderful resources for meditation. You might want to seek out a meditation teacher or a meditation group. You might also want to explore guided meditation as a form of relaxation.

It is a good idea to create a place in your home for the sole purpose of meditation. It might be a bench in an outdoor garden, or a comfortable chair in the corner of the living room. The important thing is that you do it in a place that is quiet and where you are not likely to be disturbed. But meditation can be done anywhere at any time. You might find five minutes on the commuter bus where you are able to quiet your mind and relax, or you might find three minutes while sitting in a doctor's waiting room. Yet, a routine of meditation will help lay the groundwork for a daily practice. Once you get into the habit of meditating at a set time each day, you will be able to achieve the relaxed state much more easily. You may find throughout the day—especially when life takes a negative turn—that you want to just quiet your mind. You may begin to yearn for these moments of peace after you begin to meditate on a regular basis.

Notice that when you grab for moments of quiet as a first response to an undesirable event, you are not engaging in emotional eating. Rather, you are taking a few minutes out to reset. Someone may yell at you, but instead of yelling back or allowing anger to fester, you remove yourself from the situation and regain your strength. You take a deep breath and let it out, and then you appreciate the silent, precious moment so that you will be able to return to the stressful situation with a renewed state of mind. All you have to do to put things back to normal is to stop and connect with your inner self. When you do this on a regular basis, you will lower your blood pressure, you will feel more relaxed, and you will be less likely to see food as a way to comfort yourself. You will then be able to soothe yourself in a way that also serves to bring you back to who you are at a soul level.

The benefits of meditation are multitude, but it is also important to realize that meditation is about mindfulness. Your mind is focusing on one thing so that random thoughts will not intrude. Meditation forces you to be quiet and to be able to think about just one thing. Some people use objects—a rock, a tree, a part of the body—on which to focus. You are then mindful of the one object. So as you go about your daily life, it is not a bad thing to be mindful of what you are doing. You may realize that it is better to do things slowly, and to do them right, as opposed to merely getting a lot of things crossed off of your To Do list without really getting any satisfaction from the journey. Sometimes, we try to relax by doing the opposite of achieving a meditative state. We might veg out in front of the television set, or become entranced by the popcorn bowl, or we might tune out the banter of our significant other. We are trying to relax by detaching from everything around us, but mindfulness is key to meditation and relaxation.

The next time you sit down to eat, be mindful of your environment, and of every bite of food you encounter in terms of color, texture, smell, taste and touch. Eat slowly. Focus on the food. This does not mean you need not be doing anything else while you eat. Stimulating conversation during a relaxed dinner is one of life's pleasures. Yet, when you take a bite, stop and look at the food, and when you put it in your mouth, notice how it tastes. Is it hot, cold, smooth, rough, sweet, or spicy? Does it taste good? If you find you don't like the taste, there is no reason to continue eating the food, but if it is delicious, savor the moment. Being present is the goal of meditation, and eating is the prefect time to experiment with that meditative state, even if it is for just a few seconds at a time. You may find yourself becoming more present in moments when you are eating, or just engaging in mundane tasks like braiding your daughter's hair, or walking the dog. The ordinary becomes extraordinary when we just live in the moment.

When you meditate, find a comfortable position in a quiet place. Try to arrange things so that you will not be disturbed. Wear comfortable clothing. Close your eyes. Take a breath. Create a daily practice where you meditate for ten minutes each day, preferably at the same time each day, but remember: this is your practice. Do what is comfortable for you, but do plan to devote ten minutes to meditation daily. Once you do, you will look forward to this space you created just for you. Creating a daily meditation practice helps to get you to that place where you are more relaxed, more present, and more likely to handle life's ups and downs in a positive way.

Notes

CHAPTER 12

MOVING FORWARD:
THE MAINTENANCE PHASE

This is not the end of the journey, even though you may have already shed the pounds you wanted to lose. If so, bravo! It's a great accomplishment! Some of you may still have more weight to lose but you are reading this final chapter just to see what it will be like to be in maintenance. Either way, it is important to know that maintenance is something usually equated with sameness, and while on some level that is true, it is not the whole story. We think of maintenance as the end of the road, and the end of the struggle, but life goes on. Just as you lived your life while you were losing weight, you will continue to live your life and you will continue to experience ups and downs. The difference is that now you know how to navigate life without using food as a crutch, and you also know that weight loss and weight maintenance is a process.

Think of maintenance as a place you are in when you stop attempting to lose weight. You are done with *that*. However, you need to be cognizant of what you have done here exactly, and own it. This requires a thoughtful recognition of just how much you have grown. You will recognize this, but you will continue to grow as a human being, so maintenance is really just continuing your practice of meditation, eating well and exercising.

Are You Ready For Maintenance?

How do you know whether you are ready for maintenance? This is a question that many of Sandrine's clients ask. They hang tight to the habits they created while they were losing weight. They got used to losing weight, week after week, and they enjoyed the successes. Stepping on the scale and seeing the numbers go down does feel good. But there will come a time when you are done. You will be finished with losing weight at some point, and then you will probably just replace the goal with something else. Again, what do you want to do with your life? Do you want to paint, do you want to study astronomy, do you want to go to medical school, do you want to learn to dance? Just pick another dream and it can be yours.

So, are you ready? You may be ready in many ways, but some women are reluctant to stop counting calories. They feel that they need the boundaries that calorie counting provides, and they may in fact need to count calories for several years in order to feel in control. If you feel that way, it is fine. Guidelines to maintaining your weight through calorie counting are provided in this chapter. So, are you ready now? You are if you think you are. If you begin the maintenance phase and it turns out you were not ready, go back and resume the weight loss program. If you feel that you are not ready for maintenance right now, continue with Plan A or Plan B. You may also want to ask yourself why you are considering the maintenance phase at this time. Do you want to stop losing weight because you just want a change, or do you really need to lose more weight but are not happy with the program? In other words, are you just antsy? Do you just want to do something different? Examine your goals again. You may decide to coast for a little while and then go back and lose some more weight at a later date. How you manage your weight loss is up to you, but whatever you decide, keep in mind that this is a process and your choice is always the right one.

Your Thoughts

You probably know by now that changing your thoughts leads to a change in your behavior. When you change your thoughts, the positive actions you take will come more easily. And of course, changing your thoughts requires an understanding of all of the concepts provided in this book. If you have only read this book once, read it again. Keep it on a nearby bookshelf so you can refer to it when necessary. If you find your thoughts drifting to a negative place, you have to reorient yourself to the program once again. As you move forward, and are experiencing psychological and spiritual growth, you will not need to refer to this book quite so much, but at the beginning, it is good to keep it nearby.

Maintenance: A Personal Journey

Every woman moves at her own pace. You may have truly integrated all the information from this book. You may be meditating and exercising and have lost all the weight you planned to lose, but you are not necessarily ready to let go of the calorie restrictions. You can, but you don't have to. If you want to continue to count, you can easily figure out how many calories you need to maintain your weight by multiplying your current weight by a factor of 12 through 15. For example, if you currently weigh 120 pounds, multiply 120 by 12 and then multiply 120 by 15. The result of those two calculations suggests that you should consume between 1440 and 1800 calories, dependent upon how active you are. If you exercise five days per week, use the calorie count at the high end of the scale, and if you are sedentary, you would go to the lower end. Ideally, you will be somewhere in the middle, getting regular exercise as recommended by credible health organizations. And remember, you burn calories at a rate different from anybody else. If you find you are gaining or losing weight in the maintenance phase, reduce or add calories accordingly. If you have been counting calories but want to stop while in maintenance, simply implement plan B.

If you have been successfully losing weight on Plan B already, stick to the plan. Your weight loss will level out. Eventually, when you reach your ideal healthy weight, the weight loss will stop and you can just coast into maintenance. If you find that you are still losing weight, increase the amount of food you eat. If you are exercising more than one hour each day, reduce the amount of hours you exercise. You probably never thought losing too much weight would be a problem, but the truth is that once your body experiences weight loss, it works more efficiently. Your metabolism is faster. You may find that you burn a lot of calories. And because you are no longer eating your emotions, you may actually need to eat more.

Exercise is key to maintenance because it is what will keep you healthy for the rest of your life. If you are following the exercise program in Chapter 11, implement the maintenance exercises. And remember, this is a personal journey. It is one that you create. You create the rules, you create the parameters, and while you may use this book to get there, it is all about you. You are the driver.

The Rest of Your Life Starts Now

That is all there is to know, plain and simple. You now know how to lose weight, and how to keep it off, but again, the journey turned out to be more than that, didn't it? This book has prompted you to think about things you may never have entertained before, but while thinking is a good thing, how will you use the knowledge? How will you continue your journey on a daily basis?

You may find that you are fine with maintaining your weight. You can feel what is right to eat, and you enjoy exercising. You may have signed up for your first 5K or 10K and you are reveling in all that you accomplished, but in continuing to grow, meditation is very important. It is where you find out who you are, and it is where you are able to get a glimpse at the answers to all of life's questions. Through meditation, you relax into the cosmic awareness of you, letting go of human fears, and reveling in the broader perspective you never dreamed possible. But it is possible and it is there for the taking.

Final Thoughts

This book isn't about weight loss. It is about spiritual growth. Losing weight is a by-product of that.

A point to take with you is that understanding and doing are two different things. You can go on a diet, and you can exercise, but as you learned through reading this book, the actions are different when you understand what you are doing. This book is all about changing your mind, not motivating you with veiled promises or threats—getting you excited for a while so you get off the couch or scaring you into eating healthy—as those tactics do not work. Integrating the information so it is a part of you is the most important thing you can do to change your mind. In the end, this process will only work if you do it for yourself, not for your spouse and not for your doctor, but for you alone. Eventually, if you keep on this path, you will own the knowledge. You will no longer need to use many of the tools. You know what food does to your body. You know what to eat when. And you have this book to read again and again. Losing weight is just one step on your journey to discover your true self. Enjoy the ride.

Notes

About the Authors

Sandrine Baptiste is an integrative holistic wellness coach, a personal trainer, a nutrition consultant, and the inventor of RevBall. Throughout her career, Sandrine's unique coaching style has been successfully utilized with hundreds of clients. She teaches empowering group weight-loss workshops, and lectures on a broad array of health and wellness topics.

Formerly an analyst in the insurance industry, Rhonda Tremaine is currently a versatile writer whose work appears on the Internet and in national publications. She also maintains several blogs in various subject areas.

Rhonda and Sandrine blog at www.everythingnoetic.com and plan to write more books together at ENoetic Press, the publishing company they founded in 2012.

www.ingramcontent.com/pod-product-compliance
Lightning Source LLC
Chambersburg PA
CBHW060037030426
42334CB00019B/2373